T1-Mapping in Myocardial Disease

Phillip C. Yang

Editor

T1-Mapping in Myocardial Disease

Principles and Applications

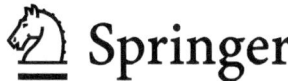 Springer

Editor
Phillip C. Yang
School of Medicine
Stanford University School of Medicine
Stanford, CA
USA

ISBN 978-3-030-08180-5   ISBN 978-3-319-91110-6   (eBook)
https://doi.org/10.1007/978-3-319-91110-6

This Springer imprint is published by Springer Nature, under the registered company Springer International Publishing AG
The registered company address is: Gewerbestrasse 11, 6330 Cham, Switzerland

Preface

Cardiovascular disease is the leading cause of death and hospitalization in the United States. Early and precise diagnosis of the cardiomyopathy will reduce the resultant morbidity and mortality from heart failure (HF). More than five million people suffer from HF with an annual incidence of 500,000 patients in our country alone. Despite significant therapeutic advances over the last three decades, the 5-year survival remains at a dismal 50%. Clinical studies have confirmed that the major sequela of HF is left ventricular (LV) arrhythmia, dilatation, and dysfunction. Patients with a history of coronary artery disease and HF have a 6-month mortality of greater than 10%, one-third of which is attributed to sudden cardiac death.

This book provides a comprehensive description of the advances in cardiac MRI to quantitate the tissue characteristics of the diseased myocardium, using myocardial and blood T1 measurements. This novel approach detects both the regional and diffuse pathological processes in the complex and contractile myocardium, the only moving organ in the human body, consisting of cardiac, interstitial, fibrotic, smooth muscle and endothelial cells. Evaluation of the native myocardial fibrosis, disarray, injury, remodeling, apoptosis and necrosis and measurement of their extracellular niche have allowed an unprecedented opportunity to elucidate the underlying pathology, provide accurate early- and late-diagnoses, and determine the prognosis of these patients afflicted with severe cardiovascular diseases.

T1-Mapping in Myocardial Disease: Principles and Applications aims to cover the broad spectrum of cardiomyopathic processes to provide a practical and meaningful guidance on how to apply this novel technique in daily clinical practice. The main objective of this book is not only to convey the innovation in T1-mapping but also to emphasize the relevance of this technique in managing cardiomyopathy patients. The specific topics include the fundamental principles of T1-mapping technique and their application in a variety of disease entities. These unique properties of T1-mapping are illustrated specifically through their ability to analyze and measure the pathology in hypertrophic cardiomyopathy, cancer chemotherapy induced cardiomyopathy, cardiac fibrosis, aortic stenosis, ischemic cardiomyopathy, uncommon nonischemic cardiomyopathy, and cell therapy for myocardial restoration. This comprehensive application of T1-mapping in cardiovascular diseases will appeal to the entire cardiovascular medicine and imaging communities.

In conclusion, I would like to express my gratitude to the tremendous effort of all the authors and the support of their family members in completing this book. I am truly honored to have experienced this opportunity to collaborate with the experts and leaders of their respective field. If I may, I would like to acknowledge my wife, Mariko, for her kind and genuine support throughout the entire duration. Her patience and unconditional support often provided the necessary emotional strength and intellectual fortitude to move forward. I also appreciate our three children, Risako, Seiji, and Masako, who challenged me to think harder, persevere and appreciate multiple perspectives, which enabled me to carry this project to completion. Finally, our pet dog, Rocky, provided sanity, calm, and many moments of self-reflection. I am forever grateful to all. Thank you.

Stanford, CA   Phillip C. Yang

Contents

Contributors

Bharath Ambale-Venkatesh Department of Radiology, Johns Hopkins University School of Medicine, Baltimore, MD, USA

Joëlle K. Barral Verily Life Sciences, South San Francisco, CA, USA

Rajesh Dash, MD, PhD Division of Cardiovascular Medicine, Department of Medicine, Stanford University Medical Center, Stanford, CA, USA

Marc R. Dweck British Heart Foundation Centre for Cardiovascular Science, University of Edinburgh, Edinburgh, UK

Russell J. Everett British Heart Foundation Centre for Cardiovascular Science, University of Edinburgh, Edinburgh, UK

Matthias G. Friedrich Departments of Cardiology and Diagnostic Radiology, McGill University Health Centre, McGill University, Montreal, QC, Canada

Kate Hanneman, MD, MPH, FRCPC Department of Medical Imaging, Toronto General Hospital, University of Toronto, Toronto, ON, Canada

W. Gregory Hundley Department of Internal Medicine, Section on Cardiovascular Medicine, Wake Forest School of Medicine, Winston-Salem, NC, USA

Michael Jerosch-Herold Department of Radiology, Brigham and Women's Hospital, Harvard Medical School, Boston, MA, USA

Jennifer H. Jordan Department of Internal Medicine, Section on Cardiovascular Medicine, Wake Forest School of Medicine, Winston-Salem, NC, USA

Yoko Kato Department of Cardiology, Johns Hopkins University School of Medicine, Baltimore, MD, USA

Christopher M. Kramer Department of Medicine, University of Virginia Health System, Charlottesville, VA, USA

Department of Radiology, University of Virginia Health System, Charlottesville, VA, USA

Cardiovascular Imaging Center, University of Virginia Health System, Charlottesville, VA, USA

Raymond Y. Kwong Non-invasive Cardiovascular Imaging, Cardiovascular Division, Department of Medicine, Brigham and Women's Hospital, Harvard Medical School, Boston, MA, USA

Joao Lima Department of Cardiology, Johns Hopkins University School of Medicine, Baltimore, MD, USA

Department of Radiology, Johns Hopkins University School of Medicine, Baltimore, MD, USA

Róisín B. Morgan Non-invasive Cardiovascular Imaging, Cardiovascular Division, Department of Medicine, Brigham and Women's Hospital, Harvard Medical School, Boston, MA, USA

David E. Newby British Heart Foundation Centre for Cardiovascular Science, University of Edinburgh, Edinburgh, UK

Mohammad R. Ostovaneh Department of Cardiology, Johns Hopkins University School of Medicine, Baltimore, MD, USA

Michael Salerno Department of Medicine, University of Virginia Health System, Charlottesville, VA, USA

Department of Radiology, University of Virginia Health System, Charlottesville, VA, USA

Department of Biomedical Engineering, University of Virginia Health System, Charlottesville, VA, USA

Cardiovascular Imaging Center, University of Virginia Health System, Charlottesville, VA, USA

Cardiovascular Division, University of Virginia Health System, Charlottesville, VA, USA

Nikola Stikov NeuroPoly Lab, Institute of Biomedical Engineering, Polytechnique Montreal, Montreal, QC, Canada

Montreal Heart Institute, University of Montreal, Montreal, QC, Canada

Yuko Tada, MD, PhD Division of Cardiovascular Medicine, Department of Medicine, Stanford University, Stanford, CA, USA

Fundamentals of Cardiac T1 Mapping

Joëlle K. Barral, Matthias G. Friedrich, and Nikola Stikov

Magnetic resonance imaging (MRI) has revolutionized the way we visualize and understand the human body. MR image acquisition enables clinicians and scientists to tweak a number of parameters (e.g., repetition time, echo time, flip angle) to generate unique tissue contrast. Each combination of parameters leads to a wealth of information about the tissue microstructure, yet reverse engineering the tissue makeup from MR images is not an easy task.

The fundamental contrast mechanisms that produce MR images are the longitudinal and transverse relaxations, characterized by the T1 and T2 parameters, respectively. The MR signal is the product of the interaction between billions of spins (atoms with a magnetic moment) over a macroscopic volume (on the order of millimeters cubed). T1 and T2 share a complex relationship, making it difficult to isolate their individual contributions to the MR signal and understand

J. K. Barral
Verily Life Sciences, South San Francisco, CA, USA

M. G. Friedrich
Departments of Cardiology and Diagnostic Radiology, McGill University Health Centre, McGill University, Montreal, QC, Canada

N. Stikov (✉)
NeuroPoly Lab, Institute of Biomedical Engineering, Polytechnique Montreal, Montreal, QC, Canada

Montreal Heart Institute, University of Montreal, Montreal, QC, Canada
e-mail: nikola.stikov@polymtl.ca

exactly how many different spin populations are being imaged, as well as what their relative contributions are.

Quantitative MRI attempts to make sense of this wealth of information using biophysical models that relate the MR signal to the tissue makeup. In this chapter we will focus on the fundamentals of T1 mapping.

T1

Hydrogen atoms (H) exhibit nuclear magnetic resonance, and water molecules (H_2O) are the source of most of the signal in MRI. We distinguish between free water, where motion is unhindered, structured water, where water is bound to a macromolecule by a single hydrogen atom, and bound water, where water is bound to a macromolecule by both hydrogen atoms [1].

In the absence of an external magnetic field, spins are randomly oriented and the net magnetization is zero. In an applied magnetic field (1.5T or 3T for clinical scanners), spins align with the applied field, contributing to a non-zero magnetization. From a classical physics perspective, spins precess around the applied field at the Larmor frequency, which is proportional to the field strength. If an ensemble of spins is now excited by a radiofrequency (RF) pulse at the Larmor frequency, the magnetization is perturbed. In a classical representation, the RF pulse

© Springer International Publishing AG, part of Springer Nature 2018
P. C. Yang (ed.), *T1-Mapping in Myocardial Disease*, https://doi.org/10.1007/978-3-319-91110-6_1

tips the magnetization away from equilibrium. The longitudinal component of the magnetization exponentially returns to equilibrium it relaxes with a time constant T1. Precession and relaxation are embedded in the Bloch equations, which describe the evolution of the magnetization over time. It is important to keep in mind that the Bloch equations are phenomenological: they agree with experience but cannot be entirely derived from first principles. They are also macroscopic, which is why we always refer to an *ensemble of spins*.

T1 is known as the longitudinal relaxation time constant, the relaxation in the z-direction, or the spin-lattice relaxation time constant. The term "lattice" comes from the early days of Nuclear Magnetic Resonance (NMR), where relaxation back to equilibrium was explained in solids in terms of interactions between the nuclear spins and the crystal lattice. We can still talk about T1 as a *spin-surroundings* relaxation time where the surroundings are the local environment of the spin. T1 relaxation occurs because of local magnetic field fluctuations due to molecular motion (tumbling) and is the most efficient (shortest T1) when the fluctuations are near the Larmor frequency, which is the case for soft tissue (structured water) but not for liquids (free water) or solids (bound water). For bound water, T1 decreases when the temperature increases because the higher temperature breaks the bonds and allows faster molecular motion. For in vivo imaging of soft tissue at common field strengths, T1 increases when the temperature increases [1]. T1 decreases in the presence of gadolinium-based contrast agents because gadolinium creates strong local magnetic field fluctuations at the Larmor frequency.

T1 Outside of the Heart

T1-weighted imaging provides an image with arbitrary units, where contrast can only be described by comparison between different tissues or with respect to a reference tissue in that same image, in a qualitative manner. *T1 mapping* produces an image, the map, in which each pixel represents the measured T1 value at that location (measured in milliseconds, see Fig. 1.7), where contrast can be described in an absolute, quantitative manner.

Fast, accurate and precise T1 mapping is never and nowhere trivial. Nevertheless, T1 mapping has been successfully used in the brain to study patients with Parkinson's disease, multiple sclerosis, stroke, schizophrenia and HIV [2]. It has yet to become part of routine clinical evaluation, partially due to the long scan times. Recently, there have been efforts to standardize the field through the implementation of vendor-specific relaxometry techniques. Cardiac T1 mapping has been leading the way in these efforts, even though cardiac and respiratory motion present major challenges. This apparent paradox might be because the arsenal of pulse sequences is more limited in the heart, making it more difficult to relate the MR signal to physiology without explicit quantification.

T1 in the Heart

Figure 1.1 shows a schematic of the composition of the heart tissue. Myocytes (muscle cells) make up 75% of the volume of the heart. The remaining 25% constitute the extracellular space, which is made of fibroblasts and collagen, other glycoproteins and proteoglycans, as well as blood vessels (smooth muscle cells and endothelial cells) [3, 4]. Each of these components has a specific T1 and contributes in a unique way to the MR signal.

Native T1

Cardiac MRI has seen tremendous growth over the past 20 years, with a recent focus put on the ability to relate macroscopic changes in the MRI signal to tissue pathology.

In the myocardium, many factors (e.g., cell volume, edema, infiltration, scarring, fibrosis) contribute to the MR signal, so it is difficult to determine the specificity of T1 to any particular spin population. Even in a single voxel, multiple

Fig. 1.1 Schematic of the heart composition

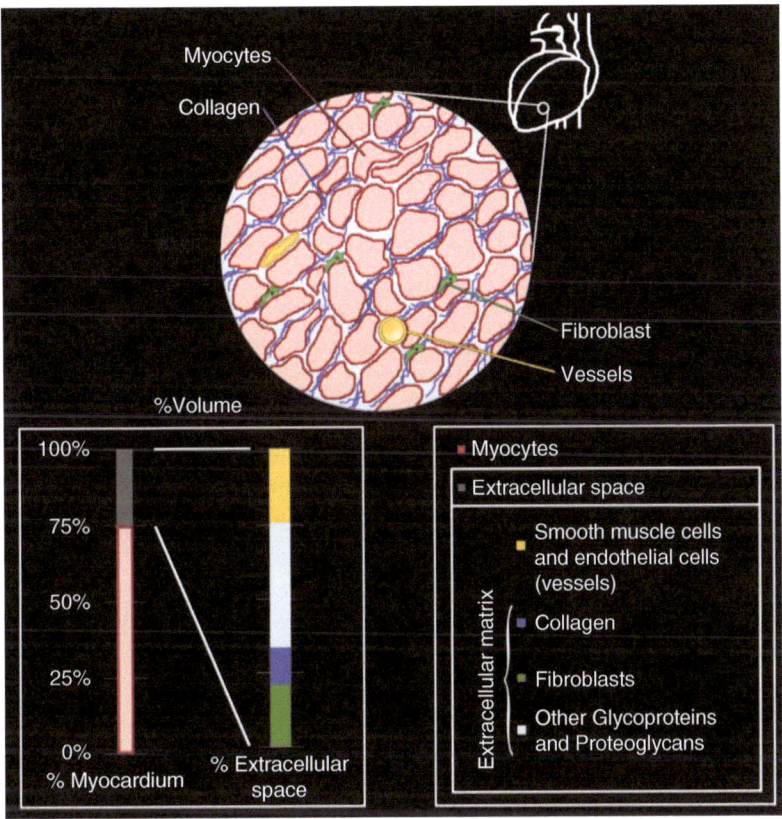

tissue compartments (homogeneous "buckets" of spins) contribute to the signal. For example, studies have explored the relationship between T1 and collagen in the myocardium of canine specimens and found a moderate negative correlation (r = −0.45) between T1 and the hydroxyproline concentration (a measure of collagen) [5]. However, this correlation is primarily driven by bulk differences in the collagen concentration between the atria and the ventricles, so it is not clear whether (native T1) can be used to discriminate between more subtle changes in collagen content that occur during scarring and fibrosis. Additionally, T1 is significantly influenced by water content, so any T1 measurements need to be controlled for inflammation and hydration.

Native T1 can still be helpful clinically, even when the underlying contrast mechanism is not fully understood. For example, recent data indicates that native T1 may allow to differentiate normal myocardium not only from acute injury with edema but also from scarring in myocardial infarction and myocarditis [6, 7]. It is also the method of choice when the risks of contrast enhancement (gadolinium side effects) outweigh the benefits. For example, contrast enhancement is contraindicated in patients with chronic kidney disease, but it is precisely these patients that are at a much higher risk of cardiovascular disease than the general population.

Late Gadolinium Enhancement

Unlike native T1 mapping that provides a narrow dynamic range in the myocardium, late gadolinium enhancement (LGE) can produce significant shortening of T1 in regions of infarction [8–10]. Gadolinium is considered an extracellular contrast agent due to its ability to diffuse from the vascular space into the extracellular tissue fluid without affecting the intracellular space. As gadolinium accumulates in infarcted tissue, it can be used as a tracer sensitive to collagen and therefore scarring and fibrosis. The decrease of T1 associated with gadolinium administration has been used to measure the extracellular volume (ECV) [11], as described below, as well as to correlate ECV with the collagen volume fraction [12].

Extracellular Volume Calculation

ECV is computed by measuring T1 before and after gadolinium administration. The difference in T1 pre- and post-contrast is interpreted as a measure of the amount of collagen present in the myocardium, because other tissues in the myocardium are not affected by gadolinium, which stays in the extracellular space. Therefore, an ECV map is physiologically relevant and easier to interpret than a T1 map. The ECV measurement assumes that the transfer rate of gadolinium between blood and tissue is much faster than the removal of the gadolinium from the blood pool. The post-contrast T1 value is highly dependent on (1) gadolinium dose, (2) time post bolus, which is hard to control in practice, (3) clearance rate, which is influenced by the cardiac output, and (4) hematocrit (ratio of the volume of red blood cells to the total volume of blood), because gadolinium is present in plasma but does not enter red blood cells. The latter is particularly important for normalizing the ECV and producing values that are comparable across patients. Recently, a method has been proposed where the hematocrit can be determined based on blood T1 [13], but it is typically obtained through an independent blood test.

In a 2-compartment model, ECV can be computed according to

$$ECV = \frac{\dfrac{1}{T1_{myocardium\ post}} - \dfrac{1}{T1_{myocardium\ pre}}}{\dfrac{1}{T1_{blood\ post}} - \dfrac{1}{T1_{blood\ pre}}} \left(1 - Hct\right)$$

where Hct stands for hematocrit.

Because of imperfections in T1 mapping, the ECV calculation is sequence-dependent and therefore difficult to standardize. In practice, however, ECV appears more robust than post-contrast T1, and it has shown prognostic value [14]. Therefore, efforts have been made towards its standardization, as evidenced by the consensus statement of the Society for Cardiovascular Magnetic Resonance (SCMR) and CMR Working Group of the European Society of Cardiology consensus statement [15]. A scientific consensus has the potential to make ECV the gold standard for the assessment of focal fibrosis. ECV can also help discriminate between non-focal expansion of the extracellular space and a sequence-dependent bias in T1, making it a candidate for evaluating diffuse fibrosis [16].

T1 Mapping Gold Standard

Inversion recovery T1 mapping was first performed in the late 1940s for NMR experiments. It consists in inverting the longitudinal magnetization and sampling it as it recovers toward equilibrium with a time constant T1. There is a consensus among researchers that gold standard T1 mapping uses inversion recovery (IR) pulse sequences with long repetition times. However, many different sequences and fitting techniques are used in practice, which can lead to a wide range of "gold standard" T1 values. This discrepancy in the gold standard makes it difficult to validate new T1 mapping sequences, as there is a large variability of reference T1 values in literature. We have investigated this problem in detail, developing a robust methodology for in vivo T1 mapping, open source code for data fitting, as well as reference data sets [17]. We expect to see additional efforts in this direction, in keeping with the concepts of open science and reproducible research [18].

The key in the development of T1 mapping techniques is to start from the Bloch equations and derive the complete signal equation keeping simplifications to a minimum. All assumptions should be stated so that further simplifications can be justified. Such simplifications are often needed to come up with a model that can be more easily fitted. Anyone using a given T1 mapping technique should ensure that the assumptions are met. For example if the model assumed TR much greater than T1, one should at least check that the value of T1 obtained is indeed much smaller than TR. This check is a necessary, but not a sufficient, condition to ensure that the model holds. The new technique should also be compared to the gold standard in simulations and phantom scans, so that expected precision and accuracy are known.

Let us illustrate this approach for gold standard T1 mapping. Consider a spin echo IR sequence

$$\left\{ \theta_1 - TI - \theta_2 - \frac{TE}{2} - \theta_3 - \left(TR - TI - \frac{TE}{2} \right) \right\} \text{ where }$$

θ_1, θ_2 and θ_3 are RF pulses, typically prescribed as 180°, 90° and 180°, respectively, TI is the inversion time, TR the repetition time, and TE the echo time. If we assume instantaneous pulses, perfect spoiling of M_{xy} after θ_1 and no off-resonance effects, then sampling the magnetization at different inversion times TI_n leads to the following data equation for the received signal:

$$S\left(TI_n\right) = e^{i\phi}\left(r_a + r_b e^{-\frac{TI_n}{T1}} \right), \text{ which has four}$$

real-valued unknown parameters (ϕ, r_a, r_b, T1). This signal equation can be simplified to a different four-parameter model if TR is much greater

than T1 or to a three-parameter model if TR is much greater than T1 and $\theta_1 = 180°$.

Model	Assumptions
$S\left(TI_n\right) = e^{i\phi}\left(r_a + r_b e^{-\frac{TI_n}{T1}} \right)$	• Instantaneous pulses • Perfect spoiling of M_{xy} after θ_1 • No off-resonance effects
$S\left(TI_n\right) = c\left(1 - \left(1 - \cos(\theta_1)\right) e^{-\frac{TI_n}{T1}} \right)$	• All of the above • TR much greater than T1 • Knowledge of the absolute timing of TI_n
$S\left(TI_n\right) = c\left(1 - 2e^{-\frac{TI_n}{T1}} \right)$	• All of the above • $\theta_1 = 180°$

Let us, for example, examine the assumption $\theta_1 = 180°$ (from the three-parameter model) a bit closer. Even if an adiabatic RF pulse is used [19], the effective flip angle depends on T1 and T2, making it impossible to obtain a perfect 180° inversion. Figure 1.2 illustrates the effects of T1 and T2 for muscle at 1.5T: the flip angle is about

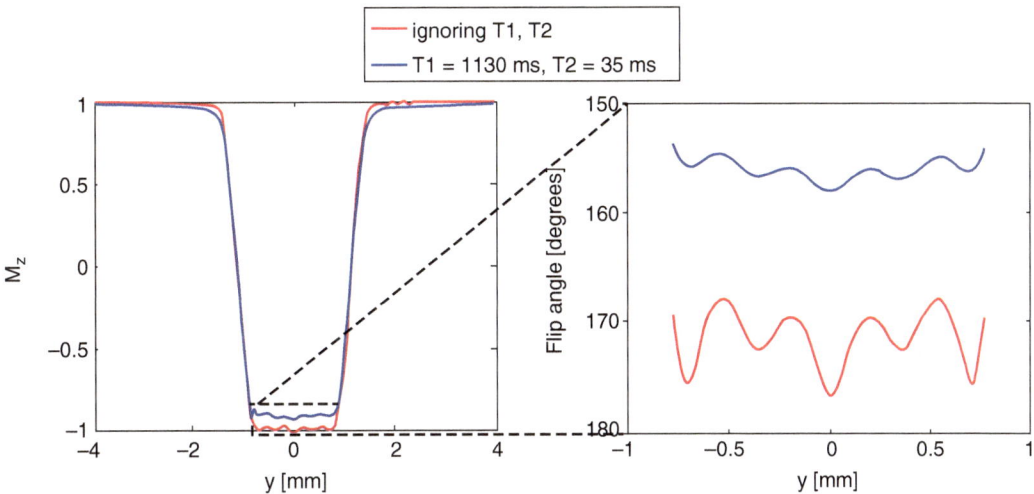

Fig. 1.2 A Silver-Hoult adiabatic inversion pulse of length 8.64 ms was simulated, with a prescribed slice thickness of 2 mm. T1 and T2 values of muscle at 1.5T were used [20]. The pulse profile is shown (left), with a zoom on the passband (right), illustrating a ~15% discrepancy introduced by ignoring T1 and T2 effects

155° instead of the prescribed 180°, which translates into the correct signal equation being

$$S(TI_n) = c\left(1 - 1.9e^{-\frac{TI_n}{T1}}\right) \text{ vs}$$

$$S(TI_n) = c\left(1 - 2e^{-\frac{TI_n}{T1}}\right); \text{ the effect is therefore far}$$

from negligible! In addition the transition bands of the inversion pulse are often partially included in the imaging slice, and the effective flip angle should be taken as the integral of the inversion profile over the slice thickness.

Once an appropriate signal equation is used, the fitting procedure should be carefully considered. Often a Levenberg-Marquardt algorithm is used and initialization of the parameters is required, which may bias the results [21]. We have proposed an alternative algorithm, which optimizes the precision and accuracy of the T1 estimation and is much faster than Levenberg-Marquardt [17]. The quality of the fit should be checked visually in different regions of interest (Fig. 1.3) to make sure that the fitting line indeed goes through (or is close to) the sampling points. Alternatively, metrics like the goodness of fit or the error (uncertainty) map can be inspected.

It is important to understand the influence of the signal-to-noise ratio (SNR) on the fitting performance. For in-vivo experiments, time is always critical and SNR is the obvious trade-off. Many sampling strategies overlook the fact that having more points on the curve may not help if each point has a lower SNR. For gold standard T1 mapping, we recommend using four points corresponding to inversion times TIs of 50, 400, 1100 and 2500 ms. One should also keep in mind that in a given T1 map the precision of the T1 estimation is worse for tissues with large T1 values.

T1 Mapping in the Heart

Figure 1.4 summarizes four T1 mapping techniques, one that is considered the gold standard (inversion recovery spin echo), and three that are commonly used for cardiac T1 mapping (MOLLI, ShMOLLI and SASHA). While there are a number of other cardiac T1 mapping sequences being developed, we focus on those that are readily available as product sequences on a clinical MRI scanner. With an inversion recovery gold standard pulse sequence, a single line of k-space is acquired every TR and TR is long (on the order of T1, typically a few seconds) to enable sufficient recovery of the magnetization before each inversion pulse [17]. For example, with a TR of 2550 ms, and a 192 × 144 matrix size (typical for a cardiac T1 mapping acquisition), a single slice gold standard acquisition takes approximately 6 min per inversion time, i.e., 6 min per point on the curve that will be fitted to derive T1.

To perform T1 mapping in the heart, both cardiac and respiratory motion have to be taken into account. If the acquisition is gated, the same phase of the cardiac cycle can be obtained every TR, and cardiac motion is less of an issue as long as the patient does not suffer from arrhythmias. Respiratory motion is mitigated by breath holding, which constrains the full acquisition (i.e., the acquisition of all the points) to be shorter than a breath hold, i.e., less than about 20 s. Another mitigation strategy is to resolve the respiratory motion either prospectively or retrospectively. If a prospective approach is taken, the sequence can be gated. If a retrospective approach is taken, one has to

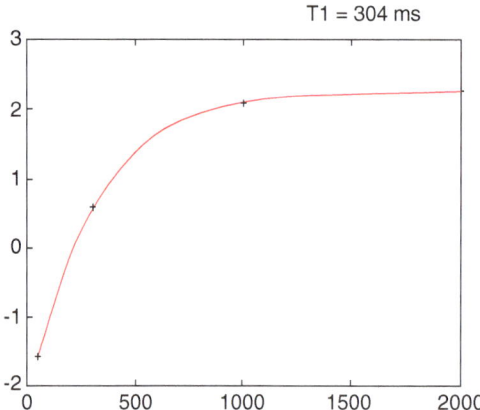

Fig. 1.3 Sampling points (blue) and corresponding fit (red) for an individual voxel in a T1 map

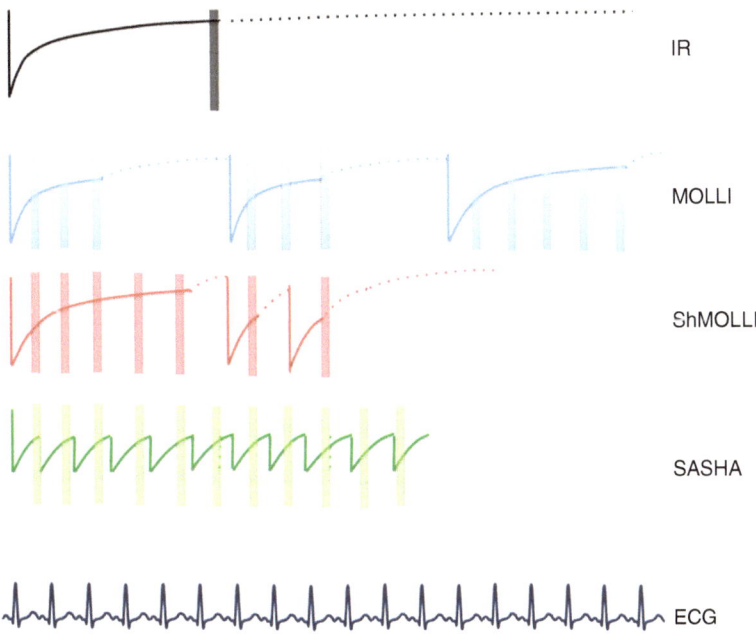

Fig. 1.4 Schematic of four T1 mapping sequences: IR, MOLLI, ShMOLLI and SASHA. The ECG signal, which is used for triggering, is shown at the bottom

either (1) ensure that k-space was fully sampled or (2) use compressed sensing or a similar technique for reconstruction [22]. Approaches combining prospective and retrospective navigation schemes have also been proposed [23].

Another challenge specific to T1 mapping in the heart is the need to be accurate over the wide range of T1 and T2 values found in blood and tissue pre- and post-contrast.

Look-Locker Techniques: MOLLI and ShMOLLI

The Look-Locker (LL) method is a rapid technique that measures T1 from a single recovery of longitudinal magnetization. It alleviates the limitation of the conventional IR method of requiring a long delay (on the order of T1) for longitudinal magnetization to recover until the next inversion pulse is played for subsequent readout. This approach was first theorized by Look and Locker and later implemented in the form of TOMROP (*T One by Multiple Read Out Pulses*) [24, 25]. The basic sequence diagram is shown in Fig. 1.4.

It consists of a single inversion pulse followed by a series of very small angle excitation RF pulses α with gradient echo readouts to sample the recovery curve. Since small angle RF pulses are used, the longitudinal magnetization is only minimally disrupted during T1 recovery and sampling is performed in a continuous manner, i.e., no wait time is necessary until equilibrium is reached. However, if the separation between α pulses is less than T2, the T1 signal is corrupted by residual transverse magnetization gathered from previous α pulses. To avoid this corruption, either the spacing between the α pulses needs to be long (>5T2), or gradient spoiling needs to be employed to crush any residual transverse magnetization. It is also important to note that due to continuous perturbation of the magnetization by successive α pulses, the recovery is driven into equilibrium more quickly, resulting in an "*effective*" T1 or $T1^*$ given by $S(TI_n) = A - Be^{-\frac{TI_n}{T1^*}}$, where the $T1^*$ calculated from the recovery curve needs to be converted to the "*actual*" T1 using $T1^* = \dfrac{1}{\dfrac{1}{T1} - \dfrac{1}{TR} \ln \cos \alpha}$ [26].

Model	Assumptions
$S(TI_n) = A - Be^{-\frac{TI_n}{T1^*}}$ $T1^* = \cfrac{1}{\cfrac{1}{T1} - \cfrac{1}{TR} \ln \cos \alpha}$	• T1 much greater than TR • Flip angle α less than $10°$ • TR much greater than T2

Recently, several variants of the LL method have been developed for cardiac T1 mapping. Basic LL cannot be applied due to cardiac and respiratory motion, so a Modified LL Inversion recovery sequence (MOLLI) has been proposed for high-resolution T1 mapping of the heart [27]. MOLLI consists of a series of single-shot images acquired in diastole, separated by inversion pulses. Several variants of the MOLLI sequence try to make the most out of a total number of heartbeats available, limited by the breath-hold duration. The first of these variants was named 3(3)3(3)5 [27]. The name indicates that three images are acquired after the first inversion pulse, three after the second, and five after the third pulse; the number in parenthesis is the number of heartbeats the sequence waits before applying the subsequent inversion pulse. Another common variant of MOLLI is the ShMOLLI sequence (where Sh stands for "Shortened"), which uses nine heartbeats (5(1)1(1)1) [28]. The last two images from ShMOLLI are used only if the T1 of the tissue of interest is short enough to allow near-complete relaxation recovery after the first inversion pulse. For longer T1s, the fitting is done only with the first five images. Note that MOLLI and ShMOLLI use a bSSFP readout and the relationship between T1 and T1* used in LL no longer holds. Empirically, the "*effective*" T1* is converted to the "*actual*" T1 using

$$T1 = T1^* \left(\frac{B}{A} - 1 \right) \quad \text{or} \quad T1 = T1^* \left(\frac{B}{A} - 1 \right) \frac{1}{\theta_1} \quad \text{to}$$

compensate for the imperfect adiabatic inversion θ_1 [29, 30].

Saturation Recovery Techniques: SASHA

Despite several acceleration strategies implemented in MOLLI/ShMOLLI, IR-based tech-

niques require long wait times for magnetization recovery. To avoid these wait times SASHA is based on saturation recovery instead of inversion recovery (Fig. 1.4). The SASHA pulse sequence images a single slice over ten heartbeats, at a specific time of the cardiac cycle. A full image, corresponding to one point on the recovery curve, is acquired every heartbeat. A saturation pulse is added and its position in the cardiac cycle varies from heartbeat to heartbeat so that each image is acquired at a different point of the recovery curve. Using a saturation pulse erases the prior history: there is no need to wait for full recovery as in inversion recovery techniques and TR can therefore be much shorter. In the original SASHA article [31], the saturation recovery times uniformly span the cardiac cycle. No saturation pulse is added before the first image acquisition so that a fully recovered image is obtained. Each image is a single-shot bSSFP image, with an acquisition window of about 175 ms. The signal equation can be written as $S = A\left(1 - \eta_{apparent} e^{-\frac{TS}{T1}}\right)$ where

- A is a scaling factor
- TS is defined as the time between the end of the saturation RF pulse and the center line of k-space
- $\eta_{apparent} = \dfrac{a}{a+b} e^{\frac{\Delta}{T1}} \eta_{actual}$ is the apparent saturation efficiency, where
  - η_{actual} is the actual saturation efficiency
  - a and b are functions of the acquisition parameters as well as T1
  - Δ is the time from beginning of imaging to center of k-space

$\eta_{apparent}$ depends on T1, therefore solving for T1 in the equation above ignoring $\eta_{apparent}$ is not exact. The assumption is that $\eta_{apparent}$ does not vary much with T1 and the dependency can be neglected.

The signal equation can also be simplified to a 2-parameter model.

Model	Assumptions
$S = A\left(1 - \eta_{apparent}\, e^{-\frac{TS}{T1}}\right)$	• $\eta_{apparent}$ does not vary much with T1
$S = A\left(1 - e^{-\frac{TS}{T1}}\right)$	• Ideal saturation

Depending on the model used, a 3-parameter or a 2-parameter fit is then performed on the magnitude of the signal intensity, with the 3-parameter fit providing greater accuracy [29]. Note that breath holding is required during the entire pulse sequence.

T1 Mapping Limitations

The table below summarizes the sensitivity of MOLLI/ShMOLLI and SASHA, respectively, to various factors [29, 31, 34, 35]. For SASHA, we only consider the three-parameter model, as the two-parameter model introduces lots of inaccuracies.

Factor	MOLLI/ShMOLLI sensitivity	SASHA sensitivity
T2	Yes, due to SSFP readout and inversion inefficiency (imperfect 180 and non-zero pulse duration)	Negligible
Heart rate and cardiac motion	Significant effect of irregular heart rate for long T1 values for which sampling occurs over more heartbeats. It can be mitigated by using a single inversion or increasing the time between inversions. ShMOLLI deals with long T1s by ignoring all but the first inversion	Long acquisition window per image (~175 ms) results in the loss of resolution
SNR	Higher SNR	Lower SNR because the sequence is saturation-based. Magnitude fit instead of complex fit introduces a bias
Off-resonance	Significant, bigger at higher field strengths and larger flip angles. ±100 Hz can result in a 6% error	Negligible. ±100 Hz results in less than 1% error
Flip angle	T1 underestimated for larger flip angles	Until SAR limits are reached, a larger flip angle increases the SNR
Inversion/saturation efficiency	Assumes ideal inversion, source of significant bias. Adiabatic pulses can help	Imperfect slice profile for the saturation, which depends on T1 and T2
Fitting model	Three-parameter fit uses magnitude data, problematic when zero crossing is close to the inversion time because SNR is low. Estimating zero crossing requires an additional parameter	Two-parameter model introduces biases, resolved when three-parameter model is used
Inflow effects (for blood T1 estimation)	More sensitive to blood flow, as it samples the recovery curve at several points after inversion. Mainly affects the longer T1s	Less sensitive as it samples the recovery curve before the non-saturated blood has flowed in
Partial voluming	Significant for small matrix size and/or large slice thickness (~8–10 mm). Blood contamination can affect the myocardium T1 estimate	
Magnetization transfer (MT)	Inversion pulses introduce significant MT effect, and T1 is underestimated	Negligible

Post-Processing

Once a T1 map is obtained, the average T1 value for a region of interest (ROI) is typically computed. Care must be taken in automating the choice of the ROI and the computation of the average T1, so that results are reproducible and no bias is introduced (e.g., due to partial volume effects from blood or epicardial fat). The choice of the segmentation method that provides the ROI should refer to published recommendations. The 17-segment model proposed by the American Heart Association is commonly used [36]. Newer methods based on machine learning look promising but most have yet to be clinically validated [37, 38]. Orientation, number of segments and nomenclature present some variability depending on the application. Figure 1.5 shows a segmental representation of the short-axis view of the left ventricle, as well as the T1 maps obtained using MOLLI, ShMOLLI and SASHA. If an observer notices artifacts (such as susceptibility artifacts), the corresponding ROIs should be excluded from the analysis. Global (averaged over the entire heart) and segmental T1 values can then be compared.

Even with cardiac gating and breath holding, motion can still be problematic, e.g., because the heart rate is variable, or patients have a hard time holding their breath. Images are often co-registered before the fit, although standard registration techniques may not work well because the different TIs lead to contrast differences. Co-registration is also used before generating an ECV map as the heart position typically moves between pre- and post-contrast acquisitions. Rather than co-registering the T1 maps, co-registration is performed on the individual images before the fit [39].

Validation

Once a new T1 mapping technique has been developed and simulated, its validation is commonly performed with phantoms and histology. Phantom validation should be the first step, and accuracy and precision can be explored using one

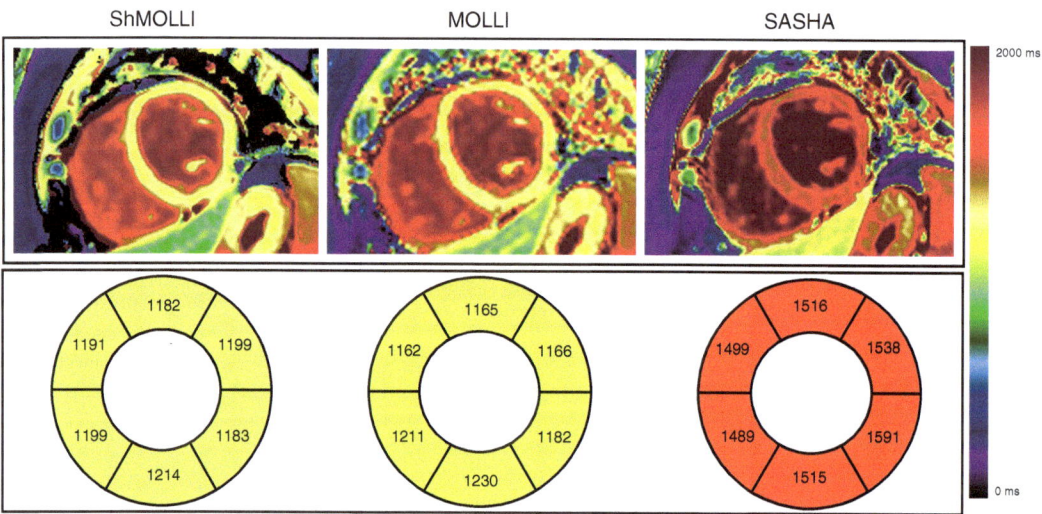

Fig. 1.5 (Top row) Representative cardiac T1 maps in a healthy subject obtained with ShMOLLI, MOLLI and SASHA. (Bottom row) Segmental analysis of the corresponding T1 maps. The details of the acquisition parameters can be found in Teixeira et al. [33]

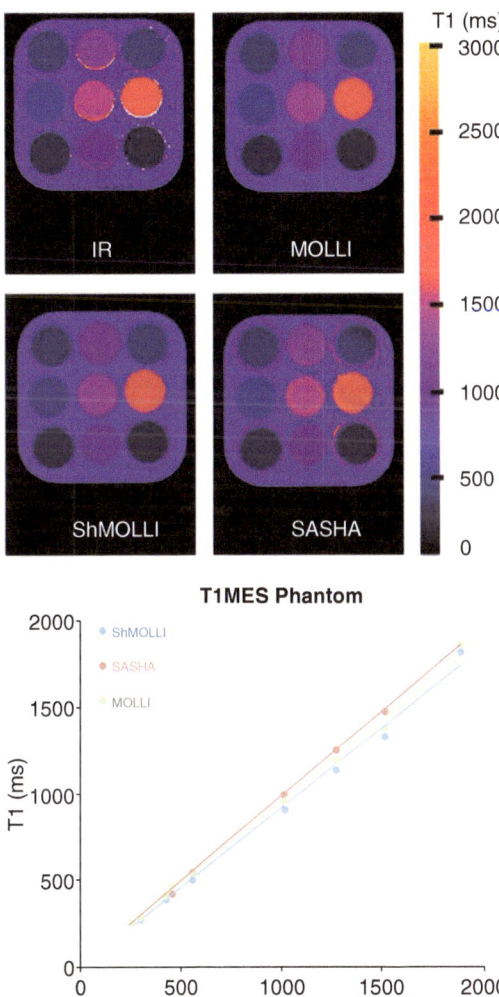

T1MES Phantom

Fig. 1.6 Comparison of four T1 mapping techniques: Spin Echo (gold standard), ShMOLLI, SASHA and MOLLI in the T1MES phantom [32]. All techniques agree well for a wide range of T1 values. The details of the acquisition parameters can be found in Teixeira et al. [33]

While most T1 mapping sequences show excellent agreement in phantoms (see Fig. 1.6), this agreement does not necessarily translate to good accuracy and precision in tissue (see Fig. 1.7). A recent study in brain MRI has demonstrated that T1 mapping sequences that agree well in phantoms can show dramatic differences in vivo [41]. These findings have recently been corroborated in the heart [33], demonstrating that in vivo T1 measurements are still confounded by magnetization transfer, RF inhomogeneity and imperfect spoiling, issues that are less prominent in phantoms. Because accuracy and precision are challenging, the focus is often instead put on reproducibility as the minimum requirement for a useful sequence. Reproducibility in cardiac T1 mapping varies but can be controlled for specific tissue/sequence parameters [42]. Precision then allows differentiating between normal and diseased tissue. From a pragmatic standpoint, systematic errors (inaccuracies) can be tolerated as long as the T1 estimate is reproducible and sensitive to pathology.

In vivo validation of T1 mapping sequences is still in its infancy. Late gadolinium enhancement remains the gold standard for non-invasive evaluation of focal fibrosis; native (i.e., non-contrast) T1 mapping and ECV make it possible to quantify the extent of expansion of the extracellular matrix and characterize diffuse fibrosis. Native T1 has been demonstrated to correlate with histology in diffuse fibrosis [43] whereas ECV has been validated with biopsy in patients with severe aortic stenosis and hypertrophic cardiomyopathy [44, 45]. Cardiac T1 mapping is still far from routine clinical use. It is primarily used as a means to observe group differences, or to provide optimal contrast for specific tissues to the radiologist. A truly quantitative approach would allow comparisons between patients, scanners, and sites, as well as across time for a given patient.

of the commercially available T1 phantoms, such as the T1MES phantom [32], or Phannie, the phantom developed by the National Institutes of Standards and Technology (NIST) [40]. Note that temperature needs to be controlled when phantoms are scanned as it influences T1.

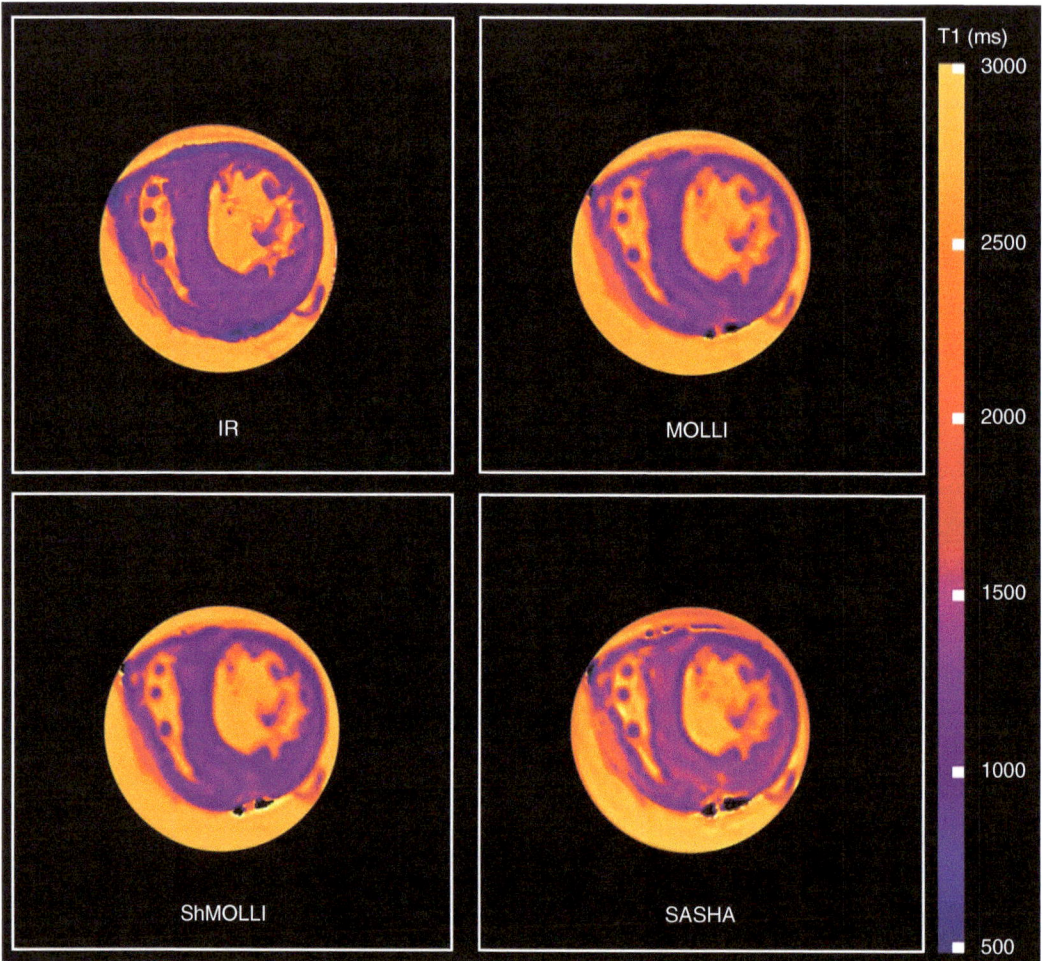

Fig. 1.7 A comparison of T1 mapping sequences in explanted pig hearts. The IR map was obtained using a turbo spin-echo acquisition and five inversion times, using a slice selective inversion pulse (TI = 33, 100, 300, 900, 2700, 5000 ms; TE/TR = 12 ms/10 s; slice thickness 8 mm; flip angle = 90°; matrix 192 × 144; FOV 360 × 270 mm and turbo factor = 7). The rest of the maps (MOLLI, ShMOLLI and SASHA) were obtained with the protocols published in Teixeira et al. [33]

Recommendations

A consensus statement on T1 mapping was recently issued by the Society for Cardiovascular Magnetic Resonance (SCMR) and the CMR Working Group of the European Society of Cardiology [15]. Regular updates by these societies are expected. A number of recommendations for performing and standardizing T1 mapping have been provided in that statement, related to terminology, scan type, scan planning and acquisition, site preparation, quality control visualization and analysis, and technical development. It is important that each site be aware of the above recommendations, to enable better standardization of T1 mapping across sites.

T1 mapping including ECV quantification is on its way to becoming an important imaging biomarker in cardiology. It has significant diagnostic and prognostic value. It overcomes limitations of signal-intensity based methods and provides unique information in diseases affecting the myocardial tissue. Current limitations include the variations and lack of standardization among sites, scanners, sequences and evaluation procedures. Even though many diseases (e.g., amyloidosis, myocarditis, Fabry's disease) have been explored by T1 mapping, data from large scale multicenter trials is lacking, and standards for data acquisition and reference values for normal and diseased myocardium will have to be established before T1 mapping can be more broadly applied. The field continues to evolve in a complex interplay between engineering progress and demonstration of clinical utility. Limitations of any existing technique have to be broadly acknowledged to make room for improved techniques that do not necessarily agree with past clinical literature.

Acknowledgements The authors would like to thank Pascale Beliveau and Tarik Hafyane for their help with preparing the figures, and Reeve Ingle for insightful discussions.

References

1. Levitt MH. Spin dynamics: basics of nuclear magnetic resonance. Chichester, UK: Wiley; 2001.
2. Tofts P. Quantitative MRI of the brain: measuring changes caused by disease. Chichester: Wiley; 2003.
3. Frank JS. The myocardial interstitium: its structure and its role in ionic exchange. J Cell Biol. 1974;60(3):586–601.
4. Rienks M, Papageorgiou A-P, Frangogiannis NG, Heymans S. Myocardial extracellular matrix: an ever-changing and diverse entity. Circ Res. 2014;114(5):872–88.
5. Scholz TD, Fleagle SR, Burns TL, Skorton DJ. Nuclear magnetic resonance relaxometry of the normal heart: relationship between collagen content and relaxation times of the four chambers. Magn Reson Imaging. 1989;7(6):643–8.
6. Hinojar R, Foote L, Ucar EA, Jackson T, Jabbour A, Chung-Yao Y, et al. Native T1 in discrimination of acute and convalescent stages in patients with clinical diagnosis of myocarditis: a proposed diagnostic algorithm using CMR. JACC Cardiovasc Imaging. 2015;8(1):37–46.
7. Kali A, Avinash K, Eui-Young C, Behzad S, Kim YJ, Bi X, et al. Native T1 mapping by 3-T CMR imaging for characterization of chronic myocardial infarctions. JACC Cardiovasc Imaging. 2015;8(9):1019–30.
8. Kim RJ, Fieno DS, Parrish TB, Harris K, Chen EL, Simonetti O, et al. Relationship of MRI delayed contrast enhancement to irreversible injury, infarct age, and contractile function. Circulation. 1999;100(19):1992–2002.
9. Pennell DJ, Sechtem UP, Higgins CB, Manning WJ, Pohost GM, Rademakers FE, et al. Clinical indications for cardiovascular magnetic resonance (CMR): consensus panel report. Eur Heart J. 2004;25(21):1940–65.
10. Wesbey GE, Higgins CB, McNamara MT, Engelstad BL, Lipton MJ, Sievers R, et al. Effect of gadolinium-DTPA on the magnetic relaxation times of normal and infarcted myocardium. Radiology. 1984;153(1):165–9.
11. Arheden H, Saeed M, Higgins CB, Gao DW, Bremerich J, Wyttenbach R, et al. Measurement of the distribution volume of gadopentetate dimeglumine at echo-planar MR imaging to quantify myocardial infarction: comparison with 99mTc-DTPA autoradiography in rats. Radiology. 1999;211(3):698–708.
12. Fontana M, White SK, Banypersad SM, Sado DM, Maestrini V, Flett AS, et al. Comparison of T1 mapping techniques for ECV quantification. histological validation and reproducibility of ShMOLLI versus multibreath-hold T1 quantification equilibrium contrast CMR. J Cardiovasc Magn Reson. 2012;14:88.
13. Treibel TA, Fontana M, Maestrini V, Castelletti S, Rosmini S, Simpson J, et al. Automatic measurement of the myocardial interstitium: synthetic extracellular volume quantification without hematocrit sampling. JACC Cardiovasc Imaging. 2016;9(1):54–63.
14. Schelbert EB, Piehler KM, Zareba KM, Moon JC, Martin U, Messroghli DR, et al. Myocardial fibrosis quantified by extracellular volume is associated with subsequent hospitalization for heart failure, death, or both across the spectrum of ejection fraction and heart failure stage. J Am Heart Assoc. 2015;4(12):e002613.
15. Moon JC, Messroghli DR. Myocardial T1 mapping and extracellular volume quantification: a Society for Cardiovascular Magnetic Resonance (SCMR) and CMR Working Group of the European Society of Cardiology consensus statement. J Cardiovasc Magn Reson. 2013;15:92. https://doi.org/10.1186/1532-429X-15-92.
16. Kellman P, Wilson JR, Xue H, Patricia Bandettini W, Shanbhag SM, Druey KM, et al. Extracellular volume fraction mapping in the myocardium, part 2: initial clinical experience. J Cardiovasc Magn Reson. 2012a;14:64.
17. Barral JK, Gudmundson E, Stikov N, Etezadi-Amoli M, Stoica P, Nishimura DG. A Robust methodology for in vivo T1 mapping. Magn Reson Med. 2010;64(4):1057–67.
18. Donoho DL. An invitation to reproducible computational research. Biostatistics. 2010;11(3):385–8.
19. Tannús A, Alberto T, Michael G. Adiabatic pulses. NMR Biomed. 1997;10(8):423–34.
20. Gold GE, Eric H, Jeff S, Graham W, Jean B, Christopher B. Musculoskeletal MRI at 3.0 T: relaxation times and image contrast. Am J Roentgenol. 2004;183(2):343–51.

21. Bevington PR, Keith Robinson D, Morris Blair J, John Mallinckrodt A, Susan M. Data reduction and error analysis for the physical sciences. Comput Phys. 1993;7(4):415.

22. Lustig M, Michael L, David D, Pauly JM. Sparse MRI: the application of compressed sensing for rapid MR imaging. Magn Reson Med. 2007;58(6):1182–95.

23. Weingärtner S, Akçakaya M, Roujol S, Basha T, Stehning C, Kissinger KV, et al. Free-breathing post-contrast three-dimensional T1 mapping: volumetric assessment of myocardial T1 values. Magn Reson Med. 2015;73(1):214–22.

24. Brix G, Schad LR, Deimling M, Lorenz WJ. Fast and precise T1 imaging using a TOMROP sequence. Magn Reson Imaging. 1990;8(4):351–6.

25. Look DC, Locker DR. Nuclear spin-lattice relaxation measurements by tone-burst modulation. Phys Rev Lett. 1968;20(21):1222.

26. Deichmann R, Haase A. Quantification of T1 values by SNAPSHOT-FLASH NMR imaging. J Magn Reson. 1992;96(3):608–12.

27. Messroghli DR, Radjenovic A, Kozerke S, Higgins DM, Sivananthan MU, Ridgway JP. Modified look-locker inversion recovery (MOLLI) for high-resolution T1 mapping of the heart. Magn Reson Med. 2004;52(1):141–6.

28. Piechnik SK, Ferreira VM, Dall'Armellina E, Cochlin LE, Andreas G, Stefan N, et al. Shortened modified look-locker inversion recovery (ShMOLLI) for clinical myocardial T1-mapping at 1.5 and 3 T within a 9 heartbeat breathhold. J Cardiovasc Magn Reson. 2010;12(1):69.

29. Kellman P, Peter K, Hansen MS. T1-mapping in the heart: accuracy and precision. J Cardiovasc Magn Reson. 2014;16(1):2.

30. Slavin GS. On the use of the 'look-locker correction' for calculating T1 values from MOLLI. J Cardiovasc Magn Reson. 2014;16(Suppl 1):P55.

31. Chow K, Flewitt JA, Green JD, Pagano JJ, Friedrich MG, Thompson RB. Saturation recovery single-shot acquisition (SASHA) for myocardial T(1) mapping. Magn Reson Med. 2014;71(6):2082–95.

32. Captur G, Gaby C, Peter G, Peter K, Heslinga FG, Katy K, et al. A T1 and ECV phantom for global T1 mapping quality assurance: the T1 mapping and ECV standardisation in CMR (T1MES) program. J Cardiovasc Magn Reson. 2016;18(Suppl 1):W14.

33. Teixeira T, Hafyane T, Stikov N, Akdeniz C, Greiser A, Friedrich MG. Comparison of different cardiovascular magnetic resonance sequences for native myocardial T1 mapping at 3T. J Cardiovasc Magn Reson. 2016;18(1):65.

34. Robson MD, Piechnik SK, Tunnicliffe EM, Neubauer S. T1 measurements in the human myocardium: the effects of magnetization transfer on the SASHA and MOLLI sequences. Magn Reson Med. 2013;70(3):664–70.

35. Schelbert EB, Messroghli DR. State of the art: clinical applications of cardiac T1 mapping. Radiology. 2016;278(3):658–76.

36. Cerqueira MD, Weissman NJ, Dilsizian V, Jacobs AK. Standardized myocardial segmentation and nomenclature for tomographic imaging of the heart. A statement for healthcare professionals from the cardiac imaging Committee of the Council on Clinical Cardiology of the American Heart Association. Circulation. 2002;105(4):539–42. http://circ.ahajournals.org/content/105/4/539.short.

37. Avendi MR, Kheradvar A, Jafarkhani H. Fully automatic segmentation of heart chambers in cardiac MRI using deep learning. J Cardiovasc Magn Reson. 2016;18(Suppl 1):P351.

38. Luo G, An R, Wang K, Dong S, Zhang H. A deep learning network for right ventricle segmentation in short: axis MRI. In 2016 Computing in Cardiology Conference (CinC). 2016. https://doi.org/10.22489/cinc.2016.139-406.

39. Kellman P, Wilson JR, Xue H, Ugander M, Arai AE. Extracellular volume fraction mapping in the myocardium, part 1: evaluation of an automated method. J Cardiovasc Magn Reson. 2012b;14:63.

40. Keenan K, Katy K, Stupic KF, Boss MA, Russek SE. Standardized phantoms for quantitative cardiac MRI. J Cardiovasc Magn Reson. 2015;17(Suppl 1):W36.

41. Stikov N, Boudreau M, Levesque IR, Tardif CL, Barral JK, Bruce Pike G. On the accuracy of T1 mapping: searching for common ground. Magn Reson Med. 2015;73(2):514–22.

42. Kellman P, Arai AE, Xue H. T1 and extracellular volume mapping in the heart: estimation of error maps and the influence of noise on precision. J Cardiovasc Magn Reson. 2013;15:56.

43. Bull S, White SK, Piechnik SK, Flett AS, Ferreira VM, Loudon M, et al. Human non-contrast T1 values and correlation with histology in diffuse fibrosis. Heart. 2013;99(13):932–7.

44. Flett AS, Hayward MP, Ashworth MT, Hansen MS, Taylor AM, Elliott PM, et al. Equilibrium contrast cardiovascular magnetic resonance for the measurement of diffuse myocardial fibrosis: preliminary validation in humans. Circulation. 2010;122(2):138–44.

45. White SK, Sado DM, Fontana M, Banypersad SM, Maestrini V, Flett AS, et al. T1 mapping for myocardial extracellular volume measurement by CMR: bolus only versus primed infusion technique. JACC Cardiovasc Imaging. 2013;6(9):955–62.

T1 Mapping in Cardiac Hypertrophy

Michael Salerno and Christopher M. Kramer

Introduction

Cardiac hypertrophy is defined as an increase in left ventricular mass and can result from a number of underlying pathologies including hypertensive heart disease, physiological hypertrophy in athletic heart, hypertrophic cardiomyopathy and infiltrative cardiac processes such as cardiac amyloidosis or storage diseases such as Fabry's Disease. The end process of an increased LV mass can result from changes in both the intracellular space due to myocyte hypertrophy and/or due to expansion of the interstitial space by fibrosis, inflammation or protein deposition. While some changes in myocardial architecture manifest as focal scar, which can be detected by conventional late-gadolinium enhanced imaging (LGE), more diffuse processes cannot readily be detected, using conventional LGE techniques. It is in this situation where techniques based on T1 mapping, such as assessment of native T1 or extra-cellular volume (ECV), can provide unique insights into diffuse changes in the myocardial structure of a thickened heart muscle. This chapter will first review the relationship between T1 parameters of native T1 and ECV with the intracellular and extracellular spaces. Then we will review the current state of the art for using these T1 mapping techniques in cardiac pathologies characterized by left ventricular hypertrophy.

Relationship of T1 and ECV to the Pathophysiology of Hypertrophy

Native T1

The native myocardial T1 relaxation time, which is the T1 of the myocardium in the absence of a

M. Salerno (✉)
Department of Medicine, University of Virginia Health System, Charlottesville, VA, USA

Department of Radiology, University of Virginia Health System, Charlottesville, VA, USA

Department of Biomedical Engineering, University of Virginia Health System, Charlottesville, VA, USA

Cardiovascular Imaging Center, University of Virginia Health System, Charlottesville, VA, USA

Cardiovascular Division University of Virginia Health System, Charlottesville, VA, USA
e-mail: ms5pc@virginia.edu

C. M. Kramer
Department of Medicine, University of Virginia Health System, Charlottesville, VA, USA

Department of Radiology, University of Virginia Health System, Charlottesville, VA, USA

Cardiovascular Imaging Center, University of Virginia Health System, Charlottesville, VA, USA
e-mail: ckramer@virginia.edu

© Springer International Publishing AG, part of Springer Nature 2018
P. C. Yang (ed.), *T1-Mapping in Myocardial Disease*, https://doi.org/10.1007/978-3-319-91110-6_2

contrast agent, is sensitive to the local microenvironment sampled by water molecules in the heart. As water is freely diffusible between both the intracellular and extracellular spaces, the native T1 measured is a weighted average of the T1 in these compartments. In this way, changes in the native T1 have a complex relationship to myocyte hypertrophy, interstitial changes, fibrosis or other processes, as well as the changes in the size of the vascular space and hematocrit. In multiple cardiac pathologies associated with hypertrophy and fibrosis (including aortic stenosis and HCM), increases in the native T1 have been associated with histological myocardial fibrosis [1, 2]. However, changes in the degree of vasodilation (such as during adenosine stress or increased afterload in AS) can also increase the native T1 [3, 4]. It is important to note that the T1 of the blood (and hence the myocardium which has a vascular volume fraction of around 10%) is sensitive to changes in hematocrit [5]. This relationship has been well described in the literature and has been used to estimate the hematocrit from blood T1 [6]. This likely explains the sex-difference in T1, which is more pronounced in premenopausal women [7]. Figure 2.1 shows example T1 maps from a normal subject, and from patients with hypertensive LVH, HCM, and cardiac amyloidosis.

Extracellular Volume Fraction (ECV)

By performing T1 mapping both with and without a gadolinium contrast agent, one can more specifically probe the fraction of myocardium which is extracellular [8]. Gadolinium is an extracellular extravascular contrast agent, which cannot distribute in the intracellular space. As the change in R1, or 1/T1, is directly proportional to the gadolinium concentration, one can measure the T1 of the myocardium and blood both before contrast and at an "equilibrium state" where the concentrations of gadolinium in blood and myocardium have nearly a constant ratio to derive the partition coefficient, lambda = [Gdmyo]/[Gdblood]. This parameter provides an assessment of the relative concentrations of gadolinium in the blood and myocardium. As the gadolinium is only distributed within the plasma space, the partition coefficient can be multiplied by (1-Hct) to determine the ECV. ECV has been shown to be elevated in hypertensive LVH, HCM, and amyloid cardiomyopathy, which are all associated with expansion of the extracellular space and has been compared to histological collagen vascular fraction [9–13]. Again, while ECV is sensitive to expansion of the extracellular space, it is important to note that it is not synonymous with myocardial fibrosis. ECV can be affected by both the changes in the interstitial space and the plasma

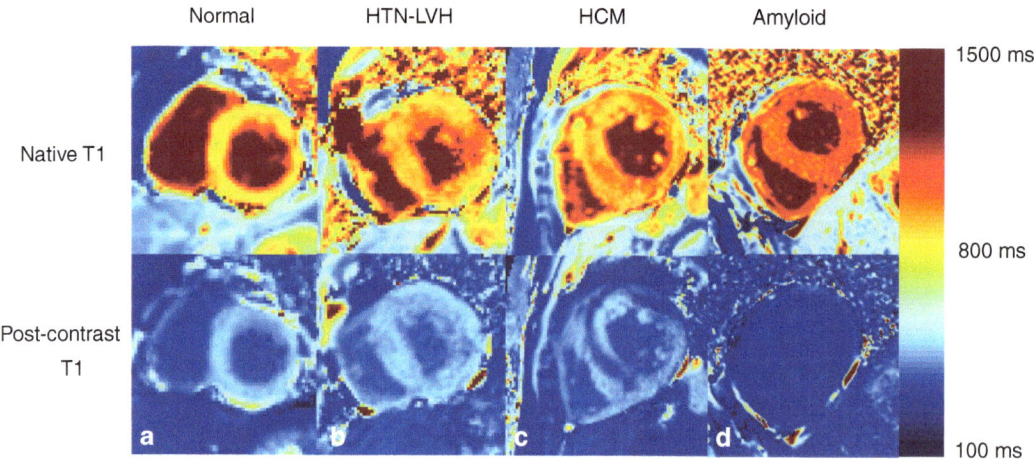

Fig. 2.1 Example Native T1 maps and post-contrast T1 maps from (**a**) a normal subject without LVH, (**b**) a patient with hypertensive LVH (**c**) a patient with hypertrophic cardiomyopathy and (**d**) a patient with amyloid cardiomyopathy. A stepwise increase in Native T1, and reduction in post-contrast T1 (indicating increased ECV) is seen across these pathologies

volume. Finally, it is important to realize that ECV is a relative metric of the extracellular space on a pixel basis. Thus, large changes in the intracellular space without significant increase of the extracellular space, or vice versa can effect ECV.

Intracellular Life-Time of Water

At high concentrations of gadolinium, which are not typically used in human studies, significant differences in T1 can be created between the intracellular and extracellular space. This is associated with the "shutter" phenomenon, which enables a two-compartment exchange model to fit the data and assess the intracellular lifetime of water, probing the size of the intracellular space [14]. This phenomenon has been demonstrated in an animal model where the intracellular lifetime of water increases in proportion with the diameter of the myocytes [15, 16]. These studies require high concentrations of gadolinium, which are typically not feasible in clinical practice, but are achievable in pre-clinical animal models.

T1 Mapping in Hypertensive Heart Disease

Hypertension is highly prevalent in the US, affecting about a third of the population, with an expected increase to over 40% of the adult population by 2030 [17]. Among adults over age 60, the prevalence of hypertension has been estimated to be as high as 65%. Hypertension is a significant cause of morbidity and mortality and about 69% of those with a heart attack, 77% of those with a first stroke, and 74% of patients with CHF have hypertension [17]. Hypertension has a significant global burden and it has been estimated that nearly one billion people in the world have high uncontrolled hypertension [17]. Patients with chronic hypertension are at increased risk of developing LVH and diastolic dysfunction [18]. In the Framingham cohort, LVH has been found to be independently associated with cardiovascular morbidity and mortality [19]. Hypertensive heart disease is associated with myocyte hypertrophy as well as with myocardial fibrosis [20]. Biopsy studies have demonstrated increased histological evidence of myocardial fibrosis in patients with hypertensive heart disease [21]. As hypertensive heart disease is a major risk factor for heart failure with preserved EF, non-invasive assessment of myocardial fibrosis could have important diagnostic and prognostic implications [22].

Several studies have analyzed changes in Native T1 and ECV in hypertension and LVH. Kuruvilla et al. studied 20 subjects with hypertensive LVH, 23 patients with hypertension without LVH, and 22 normotensive control subjects (Fig. 2.2) [9]. The study demonstrated that both native T1 and ECV (996 ± 33 ms and

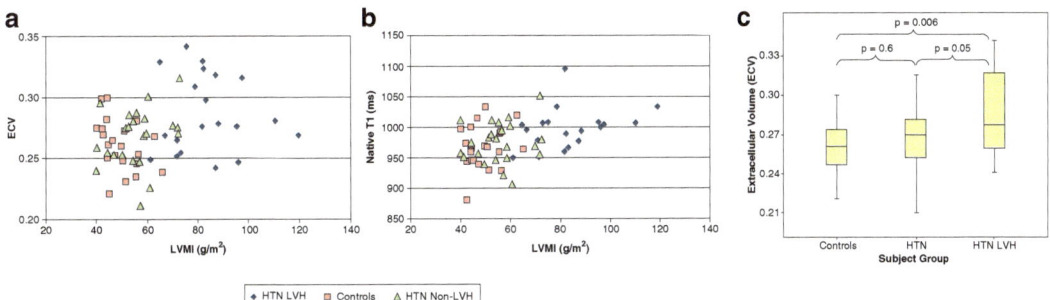

Fig. 2.2 Plot of (**a**) ECV and (**b**) Native T1 versus left ventricular mass index in controls, hypertensive patients without LVH, and hypertensive LVH (HTN-LVH). There is a modest correlation between Native T1 and ECV and LVMI. (**c**) The ECV was significantly higher in the patients with HTN LVH as compared to the controls or subjects with hypertension. There was no difference in ECV between the controls and patients with HTN. Adapted from Kuruvilla et al. JACC CVI 2015 (8):172–80 [9]

0.29 ± 0.03 respectively) were increased in patients with hypertensive LVH as compared to those with hypertension alone (974 ± 34 ms and 0.27 ± 0.02 respectively) and normotensive controls (967 ± 35 ms and 0.026 ± 0.02 respectively). However, there was no significant difference in Native T1 and ECV between patients with hypertension alone or normotensive controls. ECV and Native T1 correlated with peak circumferential strain and early circumferential diastolic strain rate. Triebel et al. performed T1 mapping and determined native T1 and ECV in 46 patients with hypertension and 50 normotensive controls [23]. Similarly, they found that native myocardial T1 was similar in hypertensives and controls (955 ± 30 ms vs. 965 ± 38 ms, p = 0.16) as was ECV (0.26 ± 0.02 vs. 0.27 ± 0.03, p = 0.06). In the subset of 14 hypertensive subjects who had LVH, there was a significantly higher ECV (0.28 ± 0.03 vs. 0.26 ± 0.02, p < 0.001). These studies suggest that there may be limits in the sensitivity of T1 mapping and ECV measurement towards detecting subtle increases in diffuse fibrosis in hypertensive heart disease before overt LVH is present.

Animal Studies of T1 Mapping in Hypertensive Heart Disease

Coelho-Filho et al. used pre- and post-contrast T1 mapping to measure the intracellular lifetime of water (τ_{ic}) to characterize murine models of cardiac hypertrophy [15]. CMR imaging was performed at baseline and after 7 weeks of either L-NAME treatment, a model which causes hypertension, cardiac hypertrophy and heart failure, or transaortic constriction (TAC) model of pressure overload. They demonstrated that the intracellular lifetime of water was correlated with cardiomyocyte size parameters such as surface-to-volume ratio and cellular volumes. Notably, in the TAC model imaged at 2 weeks, there was evidence of cellular hypertrophy that could be detected using this technique before the development of fibrosis. The authors concluded

that τ_{ic} can be used to assess cardiac hypertrophy in vivo [15].

In a follow up study, mice were randomized to either L-NAME treatment or L-NAME with spironolactone (L-NAME+S), and aldosterone antagonist for 7 weeks. CMR was performed at baseline and after 7 weeks of treatment. Animals, which had received L-NAME, had increased LV mass, ECV and intracellular lifetime of water. The animals that had also received spironolactone with L-NAME demonstrated a significant reduction in these parameters with values similar to placebo treated animals. The co-administration of spironolactone demonstrated a significant reduction in these parameters (ECV: 0.43 ± 0.09 for L-NAME vs. 0.25 ± 0.03 for L-NAME+S, $P < 0.001$; τ_{ic}: 0.42 ± 0.11 for L-NAME groups vs. 0.12 ± 0.05 for L-NAME+S group) consistent with reduction in fibrosis and hypertrophy demonstrated by histology. The animals treated with spironolactone had parameters similar to placebo animals [16].

Stuckey et al. used the murine TAC model to study diffuse cardiac fibrosis and to evaluate whether reduction of fibrosis by losartan could be detected in-vivo (Fig. 2.3). CMR imaging was performed 7 and 28 days following TAC. In this model ECV was linearly correlated with picoserius red collagen volume fraction. Treatment with losartan prevented increases in ECV demonstrating that T1 mapping techniques may be useful to track changes in fibrosis with pharmocological treatment with ARBs [24]. In the studies to date, antifibrotic therapies such as spironolactone or losartan have been given prior to the establishment of fibrosis. Whether changes in fibrosis due to antifibrotic therapies can be detected in models with established fibrosis has yet to be established.

T1 mapping in Hypertrophic Cardiomyopathy

While LGE has established itself as a prognostic marker in HCM [25], there has been growing interest in using T1 mapping and ECV to study

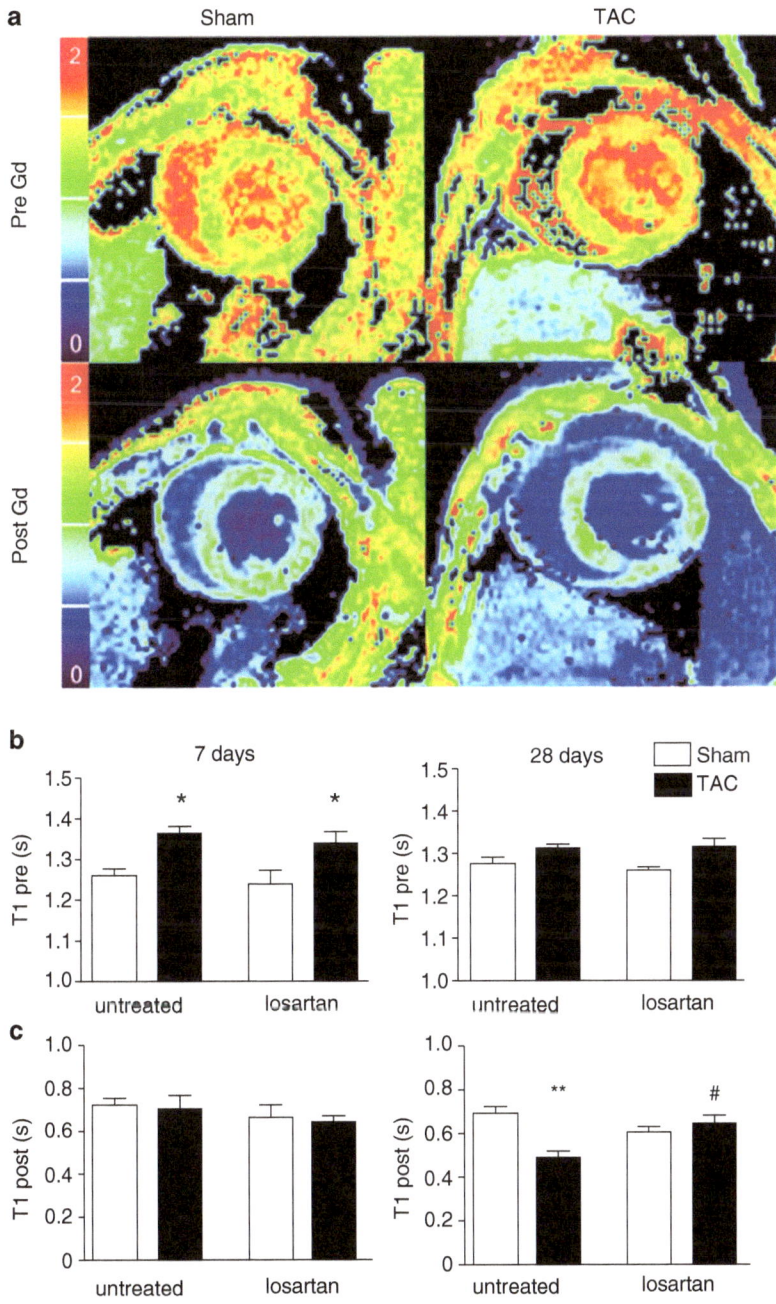

Fig. 2.3 T1 maps pre and post GBCA in a mouse transverse aortic constriction (TAC) model of left ventricular pressure overload. In the animals with TAC, native T1 was increased at 7 days both untreated and losartan treated animals. However, at this time point ECV and post contrast T1 were normal. This suggests cellular hypertrophy rather than fibrosis at early time points. At 28 days ECV was significantly higher in the TAC animals that had not received losartan, as compared to the treated animals. Modified from Stuckey et al., Circ CVI 2014; 7:240–249 [24]

Fig. 2.3 (continued)

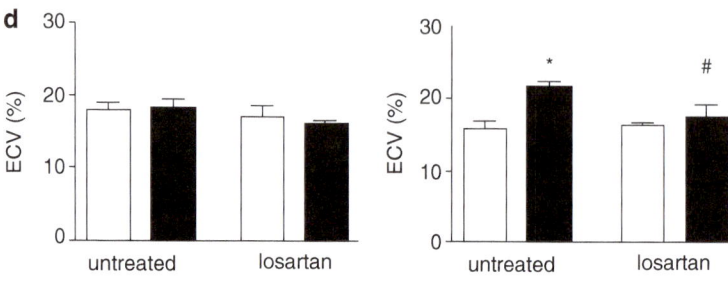

more diffuse fibrosis in HCM. Dass et al. studied 28 patients with HCM and 12 normal controls on a 3T scanner and demonstrated that the mean T1 relaxation time was increased in HCM as compared to normal subjects (HCM 1209 ± 28 ms vs. normal 1178 ± 13 ms, P < 0.05). They demonstrated that even in segments without LGE, T1 was increased in HCM as compared to normal subjects reflecting the presence of more diffuse fibrosis beyond that which is detected by LGE alone [26]. Puntmann et al. compared both native and post-contrast T1 relaxation times in 25 patients with HCM as compared to 30 normal control subjects. T1 mapping was performed pre-contrast and at 10, 20 and 30 min post-contrast to calculate ECV. Native T1 times were significantly longer and post-contrast T1 times were significantly shorter at all time-points. Similarly, ECV was increased in HCM as compared to controls. These parameters had good discriminatory capacity to differentiate cardiomyopathy from normal subjects [27]. Ho et al. used T1 mapping to determine if patients with known sarcomere mutations associated with profibrotic changes without significant LVH would have evidence of diffuse myocardial fibrosis. Ho et al. used T1 mapping to quantify ECV in 37 patients with gene mutations and LVH (G+/LVH+), 29 subjects with gene mutations without hypertrophy (G+/LVH-) and 11 healthy controls. They found that ECV was elevated in both patients with hypertrophy and those that carried sarcomere mutations as compared to healthy controls. (ECV = 0.36 ± 0.01, 0.33 ± 0.01, 0.27 ± 0.01 in G+/LVH+, G+/LVH−, controls, respectively, P ≤ 0.001 for all comparisons). This study suggested that quantifying ECV could help characterize the development of myocardial fibrosis in HCM [28].

As the presence of increased fibrosis has implications for mechanical function, Swoboda et al. evaluated the relationship between regional contractile dysfunction as assessed by feature tracking and tagging and CMR tissue characterization parameters of LGE, segmental thickness, native T1 and ECV in 50 patients with HCM. The authors found that in univariate analysis segmental thickness, native T1, and presence of ECV were significantly correlated to circumferential strain. However, in multivariate modeling, strain measurement was associated with LGE and segmental thickness but no with ECV. In a multivariate model including native T1, wall thickness and LGE, strain parameters were associated with wall thickness and native T1 but not with LGE. The authors concluded that in HCM, abnormal strain may be mediated by cellular hypertrophy, as indicated by increased wall thickness and increased native T1 rather than by expansion of the extracellular space [29].

There has also been interest in looking at the association between pro-fibrotic biomarkers and cellular markers, which are associated with fibrosis and CMR T1 mapping parameters. Fibrocytes are bone-marrow progenitor cells (BMPCs), which have been associated with multiple fibrotic disorders. Fang et al. used post-contrast T1 mapping to classify 37 HCM patient into two groups based on their post contrast T1 times as a marker of subjects with more diffuse fibrosis. Post contrast T1 mapping was also performed in 20 healthy controls. They found that the proportion of fibrocytes derived from BMPCs were increased in patients with diffuse fibrosis as compared to those without fibrosis or normal controls. The proportion of fibrocytes showed a mild inverse correlation with post-contrast T1 time (r = 0.37, p = 0.03). They also found differences in stromal cell-derived growth factor-1 in HCM patients with diffuse fibrosis as compared to those without fibrosis or to control subjects [30].

T1 Mapping in the Evaluation of Hypertrophy in Aortic Stenosis

One of the first studies, demonstrating the correlation between CMR measures of histology and ECV, was performed by Flett et al. They studied 18 patients with aortic stenosis undergoing AVR and 8 subjects undergoing myectomy for HCM. They performed T1 mapping pre-contrast and during a constant infusion of gadolinium to determine ECV. They demonstrated that the mean histological fibrosis was 20.5% in AS and 17% in hypertrophic cardiomyopathy and demonstrated a strong correlation (R2 = 0.80) between ECV and histological fibrosis [31]. Aortic stenosis is known to lead to diffuse myocardial fibrosis and prior studies have demonstrated that the presence of diffuse myocardial fibrosis is associated with adverse cardiovascular outcomes. Bull et al. measured native T1 in 109 subjects with moderate to severe AS and 33 age matched controls on a 1.5T scanner using the ShMOLLI technique and obtained biopsy samples to measure collagen volume fraction in 19 subjects undergoing AVR. The authors demonstrated a significant correlation between native T1 and collagen volume fraction (r = 0.65, p = 0.002). Mean T1 values were significantly longer in all groups with severe AS (972 ± 33 ms in severe asymptomatic, 1014 ± 38 ms in severe symptomatic) than in normal controls (944 ± 16 ms) (p < 0.05). Subjects with severe symptomatic AS had significantly higher T1 then those with moderate AS; however, there was no statistical difference in native T1 between normal subjects and those with moderate AS (955 ± 30) [1].

Whether fibrosis regresses following aortic valve replacement in aortic stenosis remains an open question. Flett et al. studied patients with severe AS both before (N = 63) and 6 months after aortic valve replacement to measure ECV. ECV was also measured in 30 normal controls. The authors demonstrated more diffuse fibrosis in patients with AS as compared to normal controls. At 6 months, a reduction in LV mass but no significant change in diffuse myocardial fibrosis suggests that the regression in LV hypertrophy following AVR may be related to reduction in cellular hypertrophy rather than regression of diffuse fibrosis [12].

Using T1 Mapping to Differentiate between Causes of Hypertrophy

There are multiple clinical scenarios where differentiating the causes of hypertrophy, using morphological features alone to differentiate between different causes of pathology. In these scenarios, T1 mapping could provide incremental information to make the correct diagnosis (Fig. 2.1).

Differentiating Hypertensive Heart Disease from HCM

While in the presence of typical asymmetric septal hypertrophy, it may not be difficult to diagnose HCM. However, it is often difficult to differentiate between hypertensive LVH and HCM with symmetric hypertrophy. Hinojar et al. performed pre-contrast and 20 min post-contrast T1 mapping in 95 patients with HCM, 69 patients with hypertension, and 23 subjects with positive gene mutations for HCM without overt disease. Native T1 and ECV were elevated in patients with HCM as compared to the gene positive subjects and hypertensive patients. Native T1 was also higher in the gene positive subjects with 65% of subjects having native T1 greater than 2SD above the normal range [13]. Thus, markedly elevated native T1 or ECV may be helpful to differentiate between HCM and hypertensive heart disease.

Differentiating Athletic Hypertrophy from HCM

It is often difficult to differentiate athletic hypertrophy from HCM. Detraining is frequently recommended for differentiation, which can have a significant negative impact on athletes. Swoboda et al. sought to determine if native T1 or ECV could help differentiate athletic hypertrophy from

HCM [32]. They studied 50 HCM patients, 40 athletes and 35 sedentary controls, using T1 mapping on a 3T scanner before and 15 min following gadolinium contrast (Fig. 2.4). Both ECV and native T1 in the thickest myocardial segments were lower in the athletes as compared to the patients with HCM (1182 ± 42 ms vs. 1261 ± 66 ms and 0.22 ± 0.03 vs. 0.32 ± 0.08 respectively). ECV was significantly lower in athletes as compared to controls (0.22 ± 0.03 vs. 0.024 ± 0.03) but there were no significant differences in native T1 between these groups. As ECV is a relative metric, it is likely that cellular hypertrophy in athletes represents a larger component of their myocardium rather than the interstitial space. Among athletes, ECV was negatively correlated with wall thickness. In HCM, there is an increase in both cellular hypertrophy and ECM deposition with a positive correlation between wall thickness and ECV. For the detection of HCM among the athletes and HCM subjects, the AUC for maximal segment thickness, native T1 and ECV were 0.986 (95%

confidence interval [CI]: 0.935–0.999), 0.847 (95% CI: 0.756–0.914), and 0.936 (95% CI: 0.864–0.977), respectively (p < 0.001 for all). There were no differences between the AUC of these techniques; however, the AUC of ECV was superior to that of LGE. This study suggests that the T1 mapping parameters could be used with maximal wall thickness to differentiate the athletic hypertrophy from HCM [32].

Differentiation of Hypertensive LVH from Infiltrative Cardiomyopathy

A consideration in the differential diagnosis of a thickened heart wall is the possibility of an infiltrative cardiomyopathy such as amyloidosis. Patients with amyloid have marked elevations in both native T1 and ECV as compared to normal controls as shown in a preliminary study by Brooks et al. in five patients with amyloid and seven controls [10]. In a larger study, Karamitsos et al. demonstrated a stepwise increase in native T1 in patients with amyloid without known cardiac involvement, amyloid with possible cardiac involvement, and amyloid with definite cardiac amyloid as compared to both normal controls and patients with amyloidosis [33]. Thus, the marked increases in T1 and ECV could help differentiate amyloid from other causes of cardiac hypertrophy.

Another group of patients, which may be difficulty to differentiate from hypertrophic cardiomyopathy or hypertensive LVH, are patients with Anderson Fabry disease. Anderson Fabry disease is an X-linked glycolipid storage disease, resulting from a deficiency of the α-galactosidase A enzyme. Patients with this disease accumulate glycosphingolipids in multiple organs, including the heart [34]. In contrast to patients with HCM or amyloid, who have markedly increased native T1, patients with Anderson Fabry disease have a marked decrease in their native T1. Thompson et al. studied 31 patients with Anderson Fabry disease, 23 controls and 21 subjects with hypertensive disease with concentric remodeling or LVH and demonstrated that patients with Anderson Fabry disease had a significantly lower native T1 [34]. Sado demonstrated that among patients with evidence of LVH, all subjects with

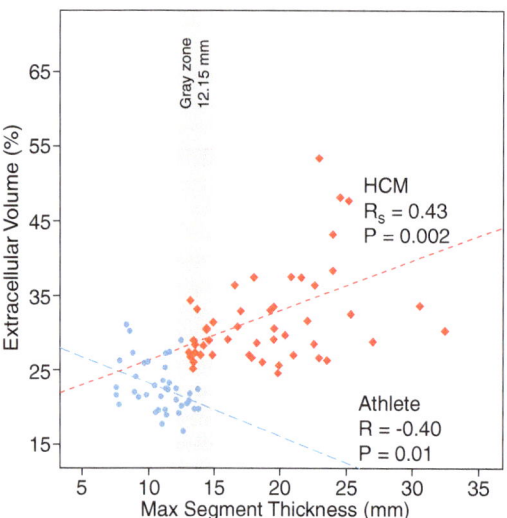

Fig. 2.4 ECV versus Maximal segmental thickness for athletes (light blue) versus patients with HCM (red). All of the athletes had a maximal segment thickness less than 1.5 mm. Within the region of 1.2–1.5 ECV and Native T1 were able to discriminate between these pathologies. In patients with HCM, as LV mass goes up ECV goes up due to expansion of the extracellular space greater than intracellular space. In athletes, ECV decreases with increasing septal thickness as the hypertrophy is due to cellular rather than extracellular expansion. Adapted from Swoboda et al. JACC 2016, 67 (18) [32]

Anderson Fabry disease had a native T1, which was less than 940 ms and differentiated this disease from patients with LVH due to hypertension, hypertrophic cardiomyopathy or amyloid cardiomyopathy [35]. Notably, measurement in the septum may be most useful as some patients with Anderson Fabry disease may have characteristic scar in the inferolateral wall, which results in an increase in native T1. As the changes in Anderson Fabry are intracellular, there is no significant change in ECV; however, this has not been exclusively studied.

T1 Mapping in Right Ventricular Hypertrophy

T1 mapping in the right ventricle is challenging using current single breath-held T1 mapping techniques due to the relatively thin wall of the RV as compared to the left ventricle. Mehta et al. developed a pulse sequence, ANGIE which uses navigator gating and advanced reconstruction techniques to obtain high resolution myocardial T1 maps (Fig. 2.5) [36]. This technique has been applied to assess patients with pulmonary

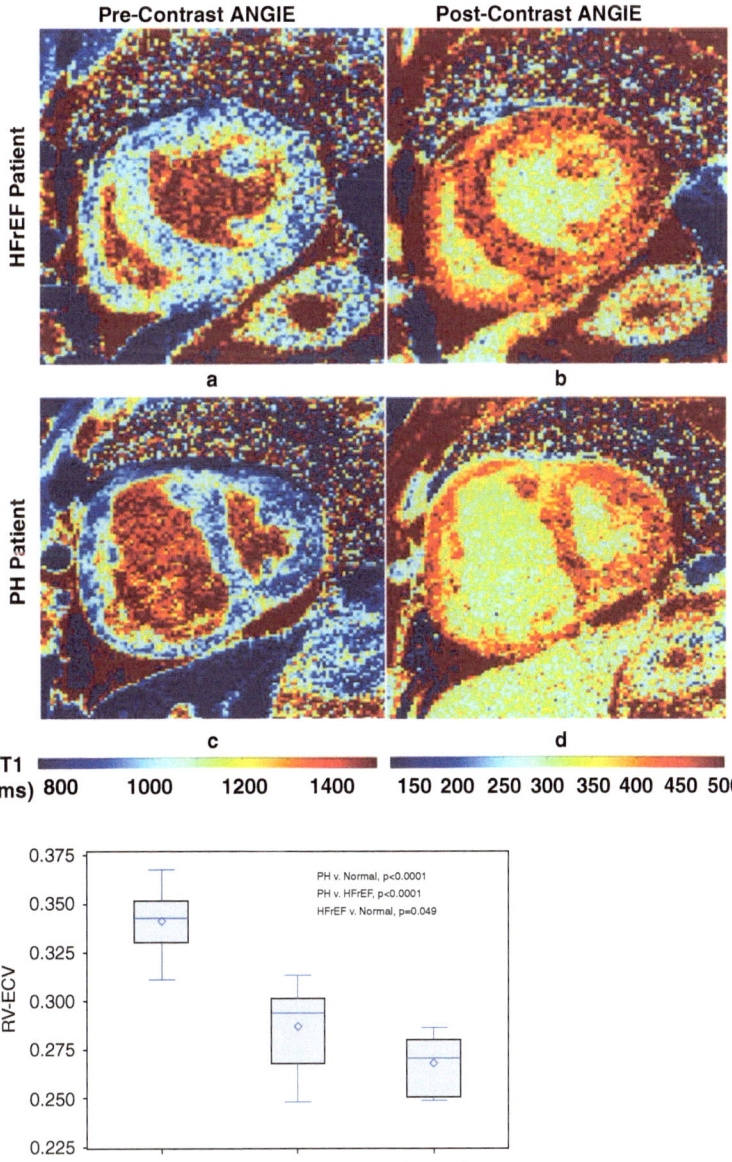

Fig. 2.5 High resolution (**a**) Pre-contrast (**b**) and post contrast T1 maps of a patient with HFrEF with secondary pulmonary hypertension and (**c**) pre and (**d**) post-contrast T1 maps from a patient with primary pulmonary hypertension (PPH) using the ANGIE pulse sequence. RV ECV and native T1 were increased in patient with PPH, and in patients with HFrEF with secondary pulmonary hypertension as compared to normal controls. Adapted from Mehta et al. JCMR 2015, 17 (110) [36]

hypertension. The authors demonstrated that native T1 and ECV are increased in the right ventricle in both patients with Type I PHTN and in patients with pulmonary hypertension secondary to heart failure with reduced ejection fraction. This could potentially serve as a prognostic marker as right heart disease is associated with adverse cardiovascular outcomes. T1 mapping could also have potential for evaluation of the right ventricle in patients with congenital heart disease.

Conclusions

Native T1 and ECV measurements can detect changes in myocardial microstructure resulting from a number of causes. Notably, native T1 and ECV do not appear to be significantly increased in hypertensive heart disease without LVH. Both native T1 and ECV are increased in hypertensive LVH; however, the increase may be difficult to detect in most patients. Patients with HCM have more significantly elevated ECV and native T1. Patients with amyloid tend to have the highest increase in native T1 and in some patients the diagnosis of amyloid may be suggested from the native T1 measurements. In amyloid, ECV is also markedly elevated; however, the presence of amyloid is typically also suggested by LGE. Measurement of ECV may not be essential to make the diagnosis of amyloid in patients receiving gadolinium-based contrast agents. T1 mapping and ECV provide unique and potentially diagnostic information in patients with athletic hypertrophy with an intermediate LV thickness of 1.2–1.5 cm. Their native T1 and ECV are decreased whereas in HCM they are increased. In patients with evidence of hypertrophy with a markedly low T1, genetic testing for Anderson Fabry disease would be indicated. Finally ECV and T1 are elevated in right ventricular hypertrophy, however, given the thinner RV wall, high resolution techniques may be required to avoid partial volume effects. Thus, T1 mapping techniques may provide innovative and valuable assessment of patients with evidence of cardiac hypertrophy to delineate the etiology and severity of the underlying disease.

References

1. Bull S, White SK, Piechnik SK, Flett AS, Ferreira VM, Loudon M, et al. Human non-contrast T1 values and correlation with histology in diffuse fibrosis. Heart. 2013;99:932–7.
2. Taylor AJ, Salerno M, Dharmakumar R, Jerosch-Herold M. T1 mapping: basic techniques and clinical applications. JACC Cardiovasc Imaging. 2016;9:67–81.
3. Mahmod M, Piechnik SK, Levelt E, Ferreira VM, Francis JM, Lewis A, et al. Adenosine stress native T1 mapping in severe aortic stenosis: evidence for a role of the intravascular compartment on myocardial T1 values. J Cardiovasc Magn Reson. 2014;16:92.
4. Liu A, Wijesurendra RS, Francis JM, Robson MD, Neubauer S, Piechnik SK, et al. Adenosine stress and rest T1 mapping can differentiate between ischemic, infarcted, remote, and normal myocardium without the need for gadolinium contrast agents. JACC Cardiovasc Imaging. 2016;9:27–36.
5. Li W, Grgac K, Huang A, Yadav N, Qin Q, van Zijl PC. Quantitative theory for the longitudinal relaxation time of blood water. Magn Reson Med. 2016;76:270–81.
6. Treibel TA, Fontana M, Maestrini V, Castelletti S, Rosmini S, Simpson J, et al. Automatic measurement of the myocardial interstitium: synthetic extracellular volume quantification without hematocrit sampling. JACC Cardiovasc Imaging. 2016;9:54–63.
7. Piechnik SK, Ferreira VM, Lewandowski AJ, Ntusi NA, Banerjee R, Holloway C, et al. Normal variation of magnetic resonance T1 relaxation times in the human population at 1.5 T using ShMOLLI. J Cardiovasc Magn Reson. 2013;15:13.
8. Arheden H, Saeed M, Higgins CB, Gao DW, Bremerich J, Wyttenbach R, et al. Measurement of the distribution volume of gadopentetate dimeglumine at echo-planar MR imaging to quantify myocardial infarction: comparison with 99mTc-DTPA autoradiography in rats. Radiology. 1999;211:698–708.
9. Kuruvilla S, Janardhanan R, Antkowiak P, Keeley EC, Adenaw N, Brooks J, et al. Increased extracellular volume and altered mechanics are associated with LVH in hypertensive heart disease, not hypertension alone. JACC Cardiovasc Imaging. 2015;8:172–80.
10. Brooks J, Kramer CM, Salerno M. Markedly increased volume of distribution of gadolinium in cardiac amyloidosis demonstrated by T1 mapping. J Magn Reson Imaging. 2013;38(6):1591–5.
11. Robbers LF, Baars EN, Brouwer WP, Beek AM, Hofman MB, Niessen HW, et al. T1 mapping shows increased extracellular matrix size in the myocardium due to amyloid depositions. Circ Cardiovasc Imaging. 2012;5:423–6.
12. Flett AS, Sado DM, Quarta G, Mirabel M, Pellerin D, Herrey AS, et al. Diffuse myocardial fibrosis in severe aortic stenosis: an equilibrium contrast cardiovascular magnetic resonance study. Eur Heart J Cardiovasc Imaging. 2012;13:819–26.

13. Hinojar R, Varma N, Child N, Goodman B, Jabbour A, Yu CY, et al. T1 mapping in discrimination of hypertrophic phenotypes: hypertensive heart disease and hypertrophic cardiomyopathy: findings from the international T1 multicenter cardiovascular magnetic resonance study. Circ Cardiovasc Imaging. 2015;8(12)

14. Yankeelov TE, Rooney WD, Li X, Springer CS Jr. Variation of the relaxographic "shutter-speed" for transcytolemmal water exchange affects the CR bolus-tracking curve shape. Magn Reson Med. 2003;50:1151–69.

15. Coelho-Filho OR, Shah RV, Mitchell R, Neilan TG, Moreno H Jr, Simonson B, et al. Quantification of cardiomyocyte hypertrophy by cardiac magnetic resonance: implications for early cardiac remodeling. Circulation. 2013;128:1225–33.

16. Coelho-Filho OR, Shah RV, Neilan TG, Mitchell R, Moreno H Jr, Kwong R, et al. Cardiac magnetic resonance assessment of interstitial myocardial fibrosis and cardiomyocyte hypertrophy in hypertensive mice treated with spironolactone. J Am Heart Assoc. 2014;3:e000790.

17. Writing Group M, Mozaffarian D, Benjamin EJ, Go AS, Arnett DK, Blaha MJ, et al. Heart disease and stroke statistics-2016 update: a report from the American Heart Association. Circulation. 2016;133:e38–360.

18. Slama M, Susic D, Varagic J, Frohlich ED. Diastolic dysfunction in hypertension. Curr Opin Cardiol. 2002;17:368–73.

19. Kannel WB, Cobb J. Left ventricular hypertrophy and mortality—results from the Framingham Study. Cardiology. 1992;81:291–8.

20. Weber KT, Brilla CG. Pathological hypertrophy and cardiac interstitium. Fibrosis and renin-angiotensin-aldosterone system. Circulation. 1991;83:1849–65.

21. Querejeta R, Lopez B, Gonzalez A, Sanchez E, Larman M, Martinez Ubago JL, et al. Increased collagen type I synthesis in patients with heart failure of hypertensive origin: relation to myocardial fibrosis. Circulation. 2004;110:1263–8.

22. Lam CS, Donal E, Kraigher-Krainer E, Vasan RS. Epidemiology and clinical course of heart failure with preserved ejection fraction. Eur J Heart Fail. 2011;13:18–28.

23. Treibel TA, Zemrak F, Sado DM, Banypersad SM, White SK, Maestrini V, et al. Extracellular volume quantification in isolated hypertension—changes at the detectable limits? J Cardiovasc Magn Reson. 2015;17:74.

24. Stuckey DJ, McSweeney SJ, Thin MZ, Habib J, Price AN, Fiedler LR, et al. T(1) mapping detects pharmacological retardation of diffuse cardiac fibrosis in mouse pressure-overload hypertrophy. Circ Cardiovasc Imaging. 2014;7:240–9.

25. Green JJ, Berger JS, Kramer CM, Salerno M. Prognostic value of late gadolinium enhancement in clinical outcomes for hypertrophic cardiomyopathy. JACC Cardiovasc Imaging. 2012;5:370–7.

26. Dass S, Suttie JJ, Piechnik SK, Ferreira VM, Holloway CJ, Banerjee R, et al. Myocardial tissue characterization using magnetic resonance noncontrast t1 mapping in hypertrophic and dilated cardiomyopathy. Circ Cardiovasc Imaging. 2012;5:726–33.

27. Puntmann VO, Voigt T, Chen Z, Mayr M, Karim R, Rhode K, et al. Native T1 mapping in differentiation of normal myocardium from diffuse disease in hypertrophic and dilated cardiomyopathy. JACC Cardiovasc Imaging. 2013;6:475–84.

28. Ho CY, Abbasi SA, Neilan TG, Shah RV, Chen Y, Heydari B, et al. T1 measurements identify extracellular volume expansion in hypertrophic cardiomyopathy sarcomere mutation carriers with and without left ventricular hypertrophy. Circ Cardiovasc Imaging. 2013;6:415–22.

29. Swoboda PP, McDiarmid AK, Erhayiem B, Law GR, Garg P, Broadbent DA, et al. Effect of cellular and extracellular pathology assessed by T1 mapping on regional contractile function in hypertrophic cardiomyopathy. J Cardiovasc Magn Reson. 2017;19:16.

30. Fang L, Beale A, Ellims AH, Moore XL, Ling LH, Taylor AJ, et al. Associations between fibrocytes and postcontrast myocardial T1 times in hypertrophic cardiomyopathy. J Am Heart Assoc. 2013;2:e000270.

31. Flett AS, Hayward MP, Ashworth MT, Hansen MS, Taylor AM, Elliott PM, et al. Equilibrium contrast cardiovascular magnetic resonance for the measurement of diffuse myocardial fibrosis: preliminary validation in humans. Circulation. 2010;122:138–44.

32. Swoboda PP, McDiarmid AK, Erhayiem B, Broadbent DA, Dobson LE, Garg P, et al. Assessing myocardial extracellular volume by T1 mapping to distinguish hypertrophic cardiomyopathy from Athlete's heart. J Am Coll Cardiol. 2016;67:2189–90.

33. Karamitsos TD, Piechnik SK, Banypersad SM, Fontana M, Ntusi NB, Ferreira VM, et al. Noncontrast T1 mapping for the diagnosis of cardiac amyloidosis. JACC Cardiovasc Imaging. 2013;6:488–97.

34. Thompson RB, Chow K, Khan A, Chan A, Shanks M, Paterson I, et al. T(1) mapping with cardiovascular MRI is highly sensitive for Fabry disease independent of hypertrophy and sex. Circ Cardiovasc Imaging. 2013;6:637–45.

35. Abascal JF, Montesinos P, Marinetto E, Pascau J, Desco M. Comparison of total variation with a motion estimation based compressed sensing approach for self-gated cardiac cine MRI in small animal studies. PLoS One. 2014;9:e110594.

36. Mehta BB, Auger DA, Gonzalez JA, Workman V, Chen X, Chow K, et al. Detection of elevated right ventricular extracellular volume in pulmonary hypertension using Accelerated and Navigator-Gated Look-Locker Imaging for Cardiac T1 Estimation (ANGIE) cardiovascular magnetic resonance. J Cardiovasc Magn Reson. 2015;17:110.

T1 Mapping in Cardiomyopathy from Cancer Treatment

Jennifer H. Jordan and W. Gregory Hundley

Cancer and Cardio-oncology

Cancer is a global health care issue increasingly requiring a multidisciplinary approach to treat the underlying malignancy and manage cancer treatment associated comorbidities. In 2016, there will be an estimated 1.69 million incident cases of cancer and more than 15.5 million cancer survivors in the United States [1, 2]. Globally, in 2012, there were approximately 14.1 million incident cases of cancer [3]. While more than a half-million deaths from cancer are reported in the United States annually, the 5-year survival rate of cancer has increased significantly over the last 30 years to an all-time high of 65.4% [4–6]. These statistics underscore the interest in addressing the comorbidities present among cancer survivors to maximize post cancer treatment quality of life and survival.

Cardio-oncology is an emerging clinical discipline that explores the relationship between cardiovascular disease and cancer treatment [7]. Mounting evidence acquired over the past 20 years highlight an increasing occurrence of cardiovascular events among cancer survivors that threatens to offset the gains achieved in

cancer treatment such that overall cancer survivorship is threatened. To understand the mechanisms by which cancer and its treatment promote cardiovascular events, recent research has focused on the use of CMR tissue characterization using T1 mapping. This technique can provide assessments of the LV myocardium before, during, and after cancer treatment. This chapter reviews the results published to date using CMR T1 mapping in patients treated for cancer with the goal of gaining understanding of the subclinical cardiovascular disease that impacts cancer survivors' quality of life and survival.

Pathophysiology of Cardiomyopathy from Cancer Treatment

Anthracycline-based chemotherapy is one of the most broadly used antitumor agents and forms an essential component of curative multidrug therapies for many childhood and advanced stage adult cancers [8, 9, 11–13]. Despite its clinical efficacy, anthracyclines (including doxorubicin, daunorubicin, and epirubicin) are associated with cardiovascular side effects. When compared to the age-matched controls, long-term survivors of childhood cancers have a 15-fold increased rate of congestive heart failure, tenfold higher rate of CV death, and a ninefold higher rate of stroke that persists throughout adulthood (Fig. 3.1) [14, 15].

J. H. Jordan · W. G. Hundley (✉)
Department of Internal Medicine, Section on Cardiovascular Medicine, Wake Forest School of Medicine, Winston-Salem, NC, USA
e-mail: jenjorda@wakehealth.edu;
ghundley@wakehealth.edu

© Springer International Publishing AG, part of Springer Nature 2018
P. C. Yang (ed.), *T1-Mapping in Myocardial Disease*, https://doi.org/10.1007/978-3-319-91110-6_3

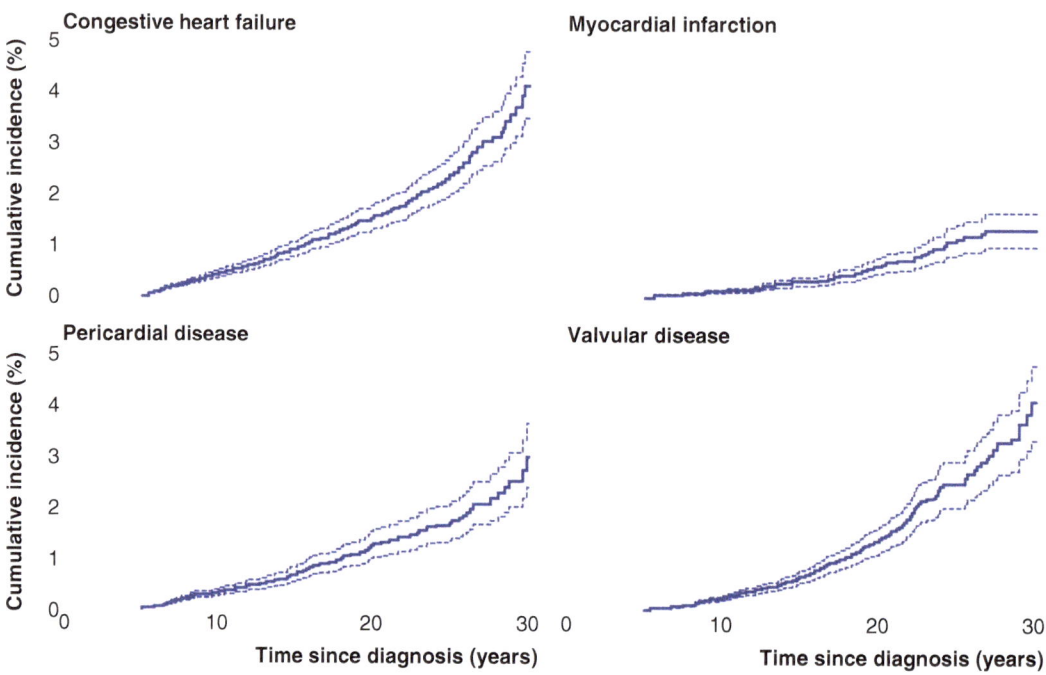

Fig. 3.1 Cardiotoxicity risk from pediatric cancer treatment continues into adulthood. The cumulative incidence of congestive heart failure (and 95% confidence intervals) for survivors of childhood cancers continues to increase into adulthood. Reprinted with permission from [14]

Survivors of childhood cancer have an 8.2 fold greater risk for cardiovascular death than normal matched controls [16]. Furthermore, the 5-year survival rate for childhood cancers has increased from 30 to 80% over the last four decades and the 5-year survival rate for breast cancer is now near 90% and steadily increasing each year [17, 18]. The prevalence of these cardiovascular events is increasing as patients sustain improved cancer cure rates. In fact, *cardiovascular events are now the leading cause of death among early stage breast cancer survivors today* [19]. For these reasons, the investigation of the etiology of subclinical and clinical myocardial and vascular abnormalities associated with the acute and chronic effects of anthracycline chemotherapy is a clinical mandate to prevent unnecessary cardiovascular events in cancer survivors.

Myocardial toxicity from anthracycline-based chemotherapy relates to the generation of reactive oxygen and nitrogen species that disrupt the cell membrane, intracellular proteins and nucleic acids that in turn modulate a multitude of regulatory pathways important in cell growth, apoptosis, and energy production (Fig. 3.2) [20]. Specifically, anthracyclines have the capability to induce myocellular death via oxidative stress or apoptosis [21]. Pathways and mechanisms for anthracycline-induced myocyte apoptosis include damage via a mitochondrial pathway from reactive oxygen species production [22, 23], DNA oxidant damage [24], and down regulation of myocellular GATA4 expression [25]. Additionally, exposure to anthracyclines can lead to the senescence and destruction of cardiac progenitor cell populations, which interferes with myocyte turnover and regeneration in the presence of diffuse cellular death [26] and may be a key contributor for the proliferation of myocardial fibrosis. Furthermore, a reduction in cardiomyocyte size from cardiac sarcomere degradation or reactive oxygen species derived from Nox2 NADPH oxidase contribute to myocardial atrophy in the setting of both cancer and anthracycline-based chemotherapy [27, 28].

Histopathologic evidence of anthracycline cardiotoxicity includes myocellular vacuolar degeneration of the sarcoplasmic reticulum,

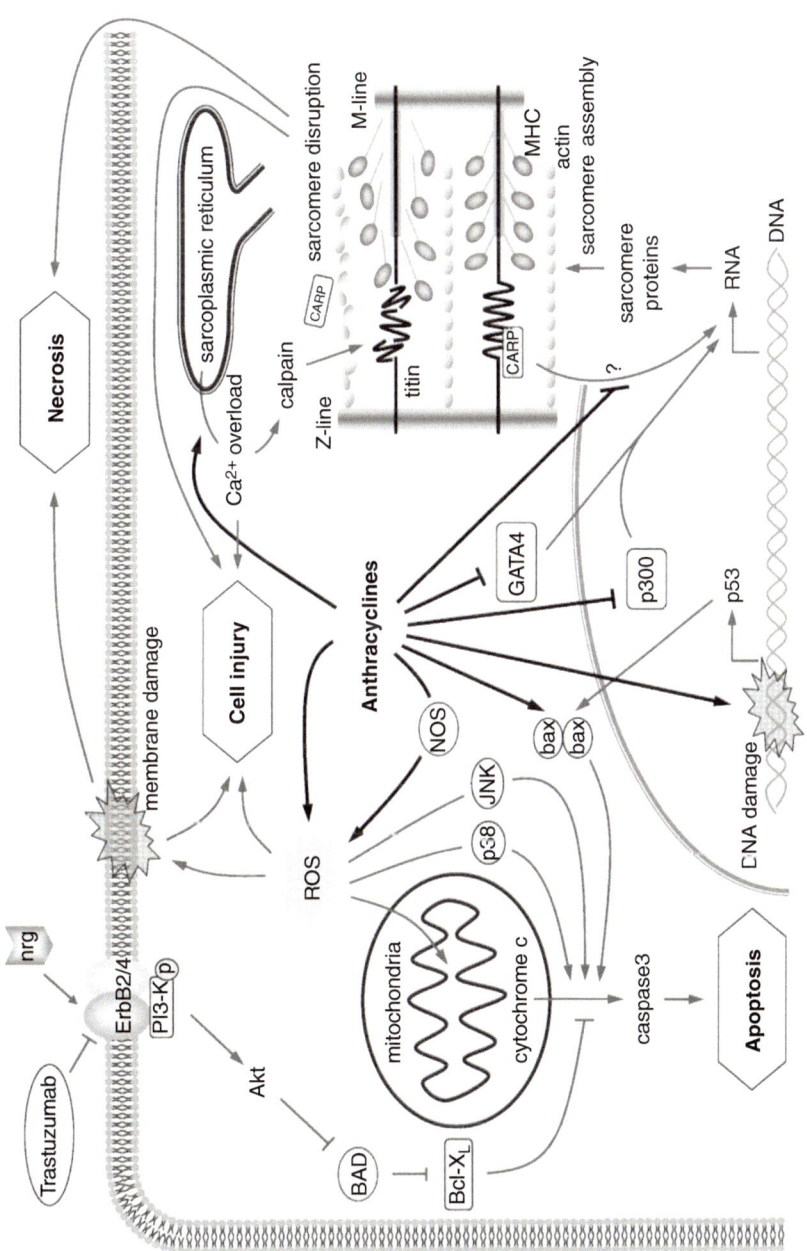

Fig. 3.2 Anthracycline cardiotoxicity mechanisms. Multiple mechanisms of anthracycline cardiac injury that promote myocellular injury and death are shown. Reprinted with permission from [20]

mitochondrial disruption and swelling, and myofilament degeneration. Each of these abnormalities precedes cardiomyocyte loss, which is then followed by replacement fibrosis [29]. Replacement fibrosis (or scar) is composed primarily of type I collagen and is the end result of myocellular apoptosis or the continued degradation of the extracellular substrate from diffuse interstitial fibrosis (from myocellular injury) that is not intervened upon [30]. Figure 3.3 demonstrates a restrictive cardiomyopathy pattern in the explanted heart of a pediatric leukemia patient treated with anthracyclines and mitoxantrone with significant diffuse interstitial reactive and focal reparative fibrosis.

The current clinical surveillance marker of cardiotoxicity is a reduced left ventricular ejection fraction (LVEF), which is a marker of global left ventricular function [31, 32]. In the setting of cardiotoxicity, a reduced LVEF occurs late in the pathophysiology and clinical presentation and is often not reversible. Therefore, it is of

high clinical interest to develop early noninvasive imaging biomarkers of diffuse fibrosis and myocardial injury that occur earlier in the pathophysiologic cascade of anthracycline cardiotoxicity. Importantly, cardiotoxicity in the treatment of cancer is not limited to anthracyclines (Table 3.1). Mediastinal and whole body radiation have been associated with coronary artery disease, constrictive pericarditis, restrictive cardiomyopathy, and fibrosis [33]. Tyrosine kinase inhibitors, such as trastuzumab for the treatment of breast cancer, have been associated with focal lesions with late gadolinium enhancement (Fig. 3.4) [34]. Furthermore, fatalities on those treated with newer immune checkpoint blockade therapies (nivolumab and ipilimumab) have been associated with fulminant myocarditis [35]. The ability to noninvasively measure early and late manifestations of cancer therapies is critical to surveillance of cardiotoxicity and evaluation of cardiovascular side effects in emerging cancer therapies.

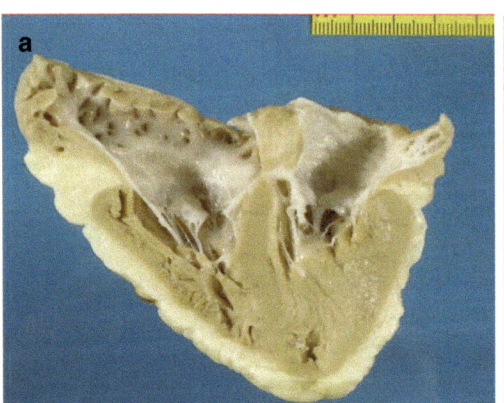
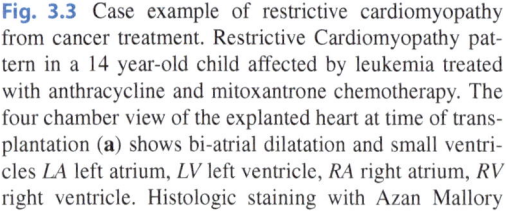
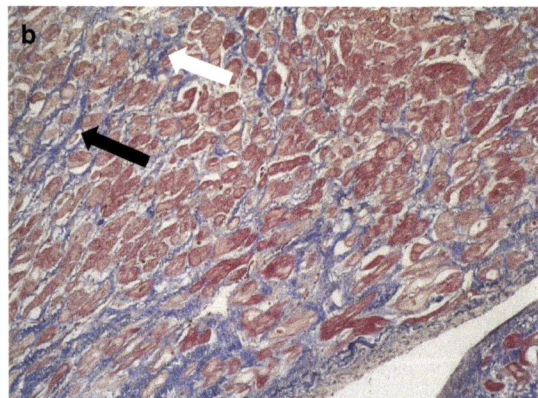

Fig. 3.3 Case example of restrictive cardiomyopathy from cancer treatment. Restrictive Cardiomyopathy pattern in a 14 year-old child affected by leukemia treated with anthracycline and mitoxantrone chemotherapy. The four chamber view of the explanted heart at time of transplantation (**a**) shows bi-atrial dilatation and small ventricles *LA* left atrium, *LV* left ventricle, *RA* right atrium, *RV* right ventricle. Histologic staining with Azan Mallory Trichrome (**b**) demonstrates cardiomyocyte anisotropy with diffuse interstitial reactive (black arrow) and focal reparative fibrosis (white arrow). Original magnification ×25. Images courtesy Annalisa Angelini, MD (Associate Professor of Pathological Anatomy, Department of Cardiac, Thoracic and Vascular Sciences; University of Padua Medical School)

Table 3.1 Cardiovascular toxicity of cancer therapeutic agents and potential utility of T1 mapping to identify cardiotoxic manifestations

Therapeutic class	Agents in class	Mechanisms	Reported cardiotoxic manifestations
Anthracyclines	Doxorubicin Daunorubicin Epirubicin Idarubicin	• *Myocellular apoptosis induction* • ETC uncoupling • Iron complexation • Lipid peroxidation of myocyte membranes • Nuclear DNA damage • ROS formation • *Fibrosis* caused by inflammatory changes	• CHF/LV dysfunction (E) • *Myocardial ischemia/ infarction (E)* • *Pericarditis/myocarditis (E)* • QT prolongation (E) • ST-T wave abnormalities (E) • *Cardiomyopathy (L)* • CHF/LV dysfunction (L)
Anthraquinolones	Mitoxantrone	• ROS formation	• Arrhythmias • CHF • *Myocardial ischemia/ infarction*
Antimetabolites	5-Fluorouracil	• Endothelial cell damage • Vasospasm	• Arrhythmias • CHF • *Myocardial ischemia/ infarction*
Antimicrotubules	Paclitaxel Vinca alkaloids Vinblastine Vincristine	• Hypersensitivity reaction • Possible vasospasm	• Bradyarrhythmias • CHF • Hypotension • *Myocardial ischemia/ infarction* • Autonomic neuropathy • Hypotension • Raynaud's phenomenon
Alkylating agents	Busulfan Cisplatin Cyclophosphamide Ifosfamide	• Coronary artery fibrosis • Hypokalemia • Hypomagnesaemia • Endothelial capillary damage • Myocardial fiber fragmentation	• Arrhythmias • Pericardial effusion • Hypertension • Pulmonary fibrosis • CHF/LV dysfunction • *Myocardial ischemia/ infarction (E)* • *LV hypertrophy* • *Hemorrhagic myocardial necrosis* • *Hemorrhagic pericarditis*
Biological agents	Interferon-α Interleukin-2	Unknown	• Arrhythmias (E) • Hypertension (E) • Hypotension (capillary leak syndrome) (E) • *Myocarditis (E)* • Thrombotic events (E) • Ventricular arrhythmias (E) • *Cardiomyopathy (L)*
Hormone-modifying therapy	Androgen-deprivation therapy Aromatase inhibitors	• Metabolic syndrome • Dyslipidemia • Insulin resistance • Obesity	• Coronary artery disease • CHF/LV dysfunction • *Myocardial ischemia/ infarction* • QT prolongation • Sudden cardiac death

(continued)

Table 3.1 (continued)

Therapeutic class	Agents in class	Mechanisms	Reported cardiotoxic manifestations
Miscellaneous	All-trans retinoic acid (Tretinoin) Arsenic trioxide Pentostatin	• Hypomagnesaemia • Unknown for many agents	• Arrhythmias • CHF • Hypotension • *Myocardial ischemia/ infarction* • Pericardial effusions
Radiation therapy		• *Fibrosis* caused by inflammatory changes • ROS formation	• Pericarditis (E) • Pericardial effusion (E) • Coronary artery disease (L) • CHF (L) • Conduction abnormalities (L) • *Constrictive pericarditis (L)* • *Restrictive cardiomyopathy (L)* • Valvular defects (L)
Tyrosine-kinase inhibitors	Bevacizumab Imatinib Lapatinib Sorafenib Sunitinib Trastuzumab	• Possible decrease in nitric oxide and prostaglandin production • *Cardiomyocyte apoptosis* • May Inhibit HER-2, EGFR, VEGF, or RAF-1 • Immune-mediated destruction of cardiomyocytes	• Arterial and venous thromboembolism • CHF/LV dysfunction • Hypertension • Pericardial effusion • QT prolongation • *Myocardial ischemia/ infarction* • *Cardiomyopathy*

This table describes the mechanisms and reported cardiotoxic effects of several therapeutic classes and agents for cancer treatment. Those that may be identified with T1 mapping methods are highlighted in **bold italics**. Modified and reprinted with permission from [32]

Table modified from Vasu and Hundley Journal of Cardiovascular Magnetic Resonance 2013, 15:66 (88) under Open Access and Creative Commons Attribution License 2.0

(E) early, *(L)* late, *EGFR* epidermal growth factor receptor, *ETC* electron transport chain, *HER* human epidermal growth factor receptor 2, *LV* left ventricle, *ROS* reactive oxygen species, *VEGF* vascular endothelial growth factor

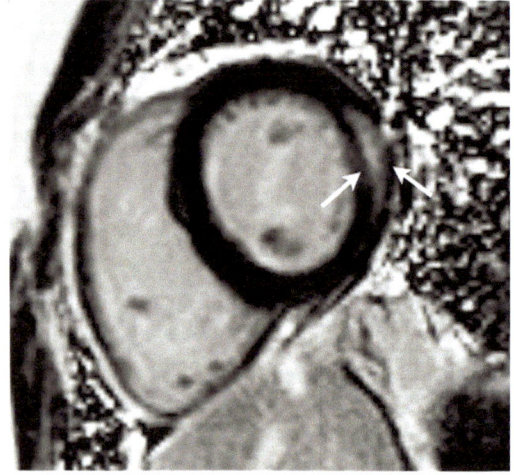

Fig. 3.4 Case example of late gadolinium enhancement in cancer patient. Mid-wall late gadolinium enhancement in lateral wall of patient with trastuzumab-mediated cardiotoxicity (arrows). Reprinted with permission from [34]

Current Imaging Surveillance of LV Function in Cardio-oncology

Left Ventricular Ejection Fraction

To date, left ventricular ejection fraction (LVEF) is the primary measure to identify myocellular injury, resulting from cardiotoxicity due to the administration of cancer therapeutics [36, 37]. The use of LVEF is particularly advantageous because it is a noninvasive imaging marker that may be measured using a variety of imaging modalities including radionuclide ventriculography (MUGA), 2D and 3D echocardiography, cardiac computed tomography (CT), and cardiovascular magnetic resonance (CMR) [38–43]. Reductions in LVEF after anthracyclines were first observed in the 1970s [44, 45], however, both MUGA and cardiac CT incorporate ionizing radiation—a limitation in those who may have additional ionizing radiation exposure for cancer treatment with external beam radiation therapy [46]. Thus, imaging modalities such as echocardiography or CMR are preferred to reduce exposure to ionizing radiation.

The diagnostic utility of LVEF in monitoring cardio-oncology patients has limitations, however, as many key therapies induce cardiotoxicity, which may manifest in other adverse injuries and events prior to a change in LVEF. These co-morbidities include valvular and pericardial disease, myocellular injury, diastolic dysfunction, and vascular injury. Patients with high grades of cardiotoxicity on biopsy can have normal LVEF measures [47] and a growing body of work demonstrates that diastolic dysfunction and heart failure may precede asymptomatic LVEF depression [39]. While current noninvasive surveillance techniques are accurate at detecting changes in LVEF they miss the opportunity to detect the early, reversible manifestations of myocardial injury after receipt of therapy for cancer [48]. Comprehensive examinations with imaging modalities should include not only LVEF evaluations but also other markers of systolic and diastolic function.

Left Ventricular Strain

A hallmark of left ventricular dysfunction in echocardiography, myocardial strain, may be measured with either 2D or 3D speckle tracking echocardiography or tissue Doppler imaging [37, 49]. Global longitudinal strain increases acutely just 1 week after anthracycline treatment from -17.8 ± 2.1 to -16.3 ± 2.0 (p < 0.01) before detectable changes in LVEF [50]. Diminished global longitudinal and radial strain measures have also been observed 3 months after anthracycline and trastuzumab treatment for breast cancer, which forecasted reductions in LVEF at 6 months [34, 51]. An early reduction of 10–15% in global longitudinal strain is predictive of LVEF decline or heart failure [52]. Changes in echocardiographic measures of diastolic function including,

decreased E/A ratio, prolonged isovolumic relaxation time, and prolonged deceleration time for early diastolic filling have been reported [53–56]; these changes, however, appear transient and their association with long term LVEF reduction remains unclear.

Serial measures of myocardial strain may also be accomplished with CMR imaging by either spatial modulation of magnetization or displacement encoding with stimulated echo CMR to measure the Eulerian circumferential strain [57, 58], however, limited data exist for serial CMR strain measures in cardio-oncology patients. Notably, however, in a prospective study of 53 individuals treated for breast cancer or hematologic malignancies with low to moderate doses of anthracyclines, circumferential strain (loss of contractility) significantly increased during a period of subclinical decline in LVEF within 1–6 months following initiation of treatment [59]. Future studies are needed to determine prognostic value of abnormal myocardial strain by CMR in cardio-oncology patients. It is important to note that myocardial strain measures (longitudinal, radial, or circumferential) can be affected by both time dependent increases in LV end-systolic volume or decreases in LV end-diastolic volume. Cancer patients undergoing therapy can experience a decrease in appetite, nausea, vomiting, or diarrhea that reduce left ventricular preload and promote decrements in LVEF and myocardial strain [60]. Therefore, when assessing myocardial strain, simultaneous assessments of LV volumes should also be performed so that strain changes may be interpreted while simultaneously considering LV volumes [61, 62].

Evaluation of cardiovascular dysfunction by markers of LV volumes, LVEF, and strain may be performed with a variety of imaging modalities with increasingly high reproducibility and accuracy, however, these imaging parameters are unable to distinguish the underlying cause of dysfunction. Cardiovascular magnetic resonance with tissue characterization techniques such as T1 mapping may be able to define the etiology of cardiovascular dysfunction in cardio-oncology patients at risk for cardiovascular events.

T1 Mapping in Cardio-oncology

T1 mapping reflects intra- and extra-cellular myopathy including inflammation, edema, and fibrosis (see Chap. 1) that are included in the spectrum of cardiotoxicity from cancer treatments. This section reviews the historical evidence of T1 changes in cardiomyopathy from cancer treatment through evolving imaging methodologies and application to the field to identify myocardial injury and fibrosis through semi-quantitative and quantitative methods.

Myocardial Injury

While current noninvasive surveillance techniques are accurate at detecting changes in LVEF, they miss the opportunity to detect the early, reversible manifestations of myocardial injury after receipt of doxorubicin [48, 63]. Studies from the 1970s demonstrated that intracellular and extracellular myocardial edema are early manifestations of cardiac injury that occur before myocellular death, increased collagen deposition, reduced contractile performance, and left ventricular remodeling [64, 65]. Spectroscopy and nuclear magnetic resonance used in rodent studies of cardiotoxicity demonstrated an increase in myocardial T1 of rodents with histological evidence of myocardial injury and cardiotoxicity [66, 67].

Following these spectroscopic observations of T1 changes, several semi-quantitative T1-weighted CMR studies using early and late gadolinium enhancement were performed. In clinically stable patients treated with anthracyclines and imaged serially with early enhancement T1-weighted CMR, a relative enhancement >5 on day 3 predicted a significant decline in LVEF at day 28 [68]. Similarly, mean signal intensity of the myocardium on late gadolinium enhancement images predicted declines in LVEF in a rodent model of doxorubicin cardiotoxicity [69]. As demonstrated in the histopathology in Fig. 3.5, the increase in mean late gadolinium enhancement T1-weighted signal intensity of

doxorubicin-treated animals with LVEF drops was associated with vacuolization. These early serial changes in late gadolinium enhancement T1-weighted signal intensity were then replicated in a clinical population as early as 3 months after initiation of chemotherapy [70]. Following these and other studies, newer quantitative mapping techniques became available to resolve limitations of T1-weighted imaging that identified myocardial changes but could not discriminate well between acute injury and myocardial fibrosis and were difficult to perform in multi-center clinical designs due to scanner variability.

Myocardial Fibrosis

Though published quantitative T1 mapping data in the field of cardio-oncology is limited, the utility of noninvasive tissue characterization in this population with complex, heterogeneous underlying risk factors for extracellular and intracellular pathologies is promising particularly given the myriad of cardiovascular consequences of therapies (Table 3.2). Studies have identified the correlation of collagen volume fraction with CMR measures of extracellular volume (see Chap. 1) and the ability to perform T1 mapping with and without contrast discriminates between intra- and extra-cellular processes. Cancer treatments may involve complex treatments such as radiation therapy followed by anthracycline chemotherapy, each with independent risk of developing myocardial fibrosis (Fig. 3.6). Thus, T1 and ECV mapping with CMR offers the ability to noninvasively perform serial assessments of the myocardial substrate, particularly in those at high risk or with underlying cardiovascular comorbidities that may contribute to baseline increases in extracellular volume. Myocardial fibrosis may be the new frontier in cardiotoxicity and thus, CMR with T1 and ECV is well poised for application in this population [10].

In a cross-sectional study of symptomatic adult survivors treated with anthracycline chemotherapy who later underwent clinically indicated 3T CMR examinations (89 ± 40 months), ECV

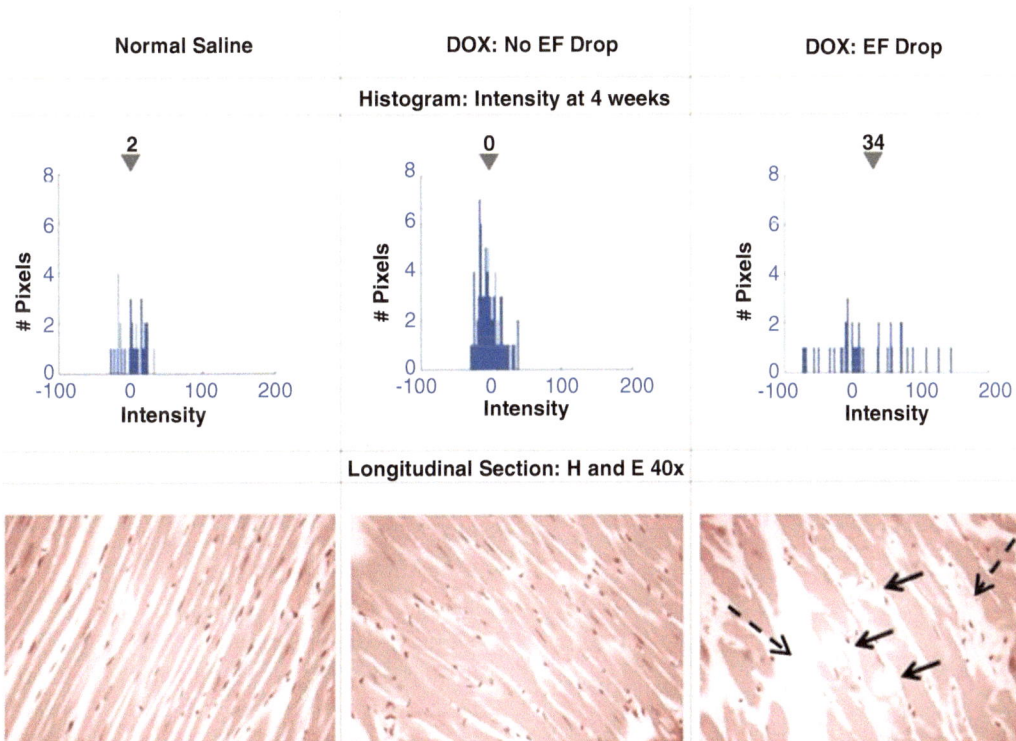

Fig. 3.5 Serial histograms and histopathology of changes in myocardial tissue following administration of chemotherapy with qualitative CMR imaging. Four week histograms of the number of pixels (y axes) and intensities (x axes) in individual animals after receipt of normal saline (top left), doxorubicin (DOX) without an EF drop (top middle), and DOX with an EF drop (top right). Increases in signal intensity represent contrast enhancement in areas of myopathy. The bottom row displays 40× hematoxylin and eosin histopathologic images from the same animals. The increased mean intensity in the animals with an LVEF drop corresponds with vacuolization (arrows, bottom right) and increased extracellular volume (dashed arrows, bottom right) on histologic images. Reprinted with permission from [69]

Table 3.2 Cardiac lesions associated with cancer therapies

Interstitial	Myocellular	Intramyocardial vascular
Diffuse interstitial fibrosis	Myofibrillar loss	Vessel thickening
Reparative fibrosis	Vacuolizations	Endothelial injury
Perivascular fibrosis	Necrosis	Perivascular fibrosis
	Apoptosis	
	Chromatin condensation	
	Picknotic nuceli	

This table lists cardiac lesions that may occur after cancer therapy administration categorized by location, many of which may contribute to changes in T1 values in cancer patients

was elevated compared to healthy controls (36 ± 3%, p < 0.0001) [71]. Furthermore, the ECV was highest among survivors with reduced LVEF compared to survivors with preserved LVEF (38 ± 3% vs. 36 ± 2%, p = 0.03), suggesting that there may be a stepwise progression of ECV with respect to LVEF reduction and increased ECV and myocardial fibrosis may precede LVEF reductions (Fig. 3.7). In pediatric survivor populations 7–10 years after treatment with anthracyclines, T1 and ECV have measured in the normal range in aggregate, however, a small proportion of asymptomatic subjects exhibited

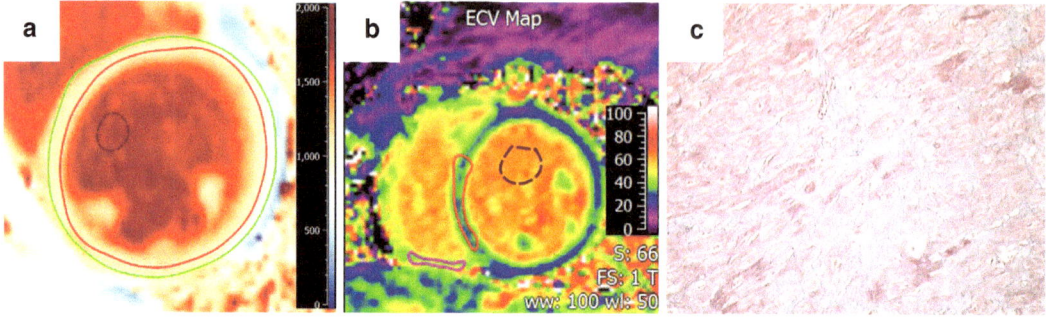

Fig. 3.6 Case example of diffuse myocardial fibrosis with T1 mapping and elevated ECV in cancer survivor. A 40 year old female treated 14 years prior with whole body radiation and three courses of high dose anthracycline-based chemotherapy. The patient had LV systolic dysfunction (LVEF 39%) with no evidence of late gadolinium enhancement using CMR imaging. As shown in (**a**), the Native T1 was homogenously elevated (>1000 ms) and both septal and right ventricular extracellular volume were also elevated at 38% and 45%, respectively (**b**). Tissue histology after heart transplantation for intractable right heart failure revealed extensive fine interstitial fibrosis (black arrows) around myocytes (white arrows) by Masson's trichome stain (**c**). Images courtesy Matthias Schmitt, MD, PhD (North West Heart Centre, University Hospital of South Manchester)

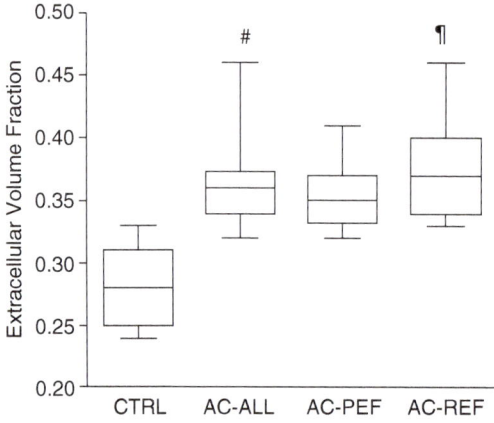

Fig. 3.7 Extracellular volume fraction is elevated in anthracycline-treated cancer survivors. Aggregate mean and ranges of myocardial ECV in healthy controls (CTRL) and patients with previous anthracycline treatment (AC-ALL). Survivors (AC-ALL) were then divided into with preserved LVEF (AC-PEF) and those with reduced LVEF (AC-REF). ECV was elevated in AC-ALL compared to healthy CTRL participants (#p < 0.001). Furthermore, ECV was higher in those with reduced LVEF (AC-REF) than those with preserved LVEF (AC-PEF) (¶p = 0.03). Reprinted with permission from [71]

T1 and ECV are elevated in anthracycline-treated cancer survivors earlier (2 years after treatment) and elevations in T1 and ECV are independent of other factors that may contribute to myocardial fibrosis including age, gender, cardiovascular risk factors, and LV remodeling parameters (Fig. 3.9) [74]. These study results demonstrate the incremental effect of anthracyclines on development of myocardial fibrosis that can be identified noninvasively with T1 mapping (Fig. 3.10). Moreover, anthracycline-induced myocardial fibrosis has been observed in serial imaging as early as 3 months after initiation of chemotherapy (Fig. 3.11) [75], suggesting the need for potential early surveillance using T1 mapping within CMR protocols as shown in Table 3.3 for assessment of left ventricular function and tissue characterization in cardio-oncology patients. In a recent animal model, early edema and fibrosis were strongly associated with and was predictive of late mortality [76]; these findings, however, have not been replicated yet in a longitudinal clinical study. Several studies addressing the NIH cardiotoxicity workshop recommendations are actively investigating the development of myocardial fibrosis and its relationship with late outcomes including, LV dysfunction, fatigue, and reduced exercise capacity previously observed in cardio-oncology populations [77].

elevated ECV similar to adult survivors (38 ± 7%) [72, 73]. Interestingly, increased ECV correlated with increased cumulative dose of anthracyclines, reduced exercise capacity (peak VO2), and LV remodeling measures (Fig. 3.8).

More recent findings using T1 mapping in the cardio-oncology setting have shown that

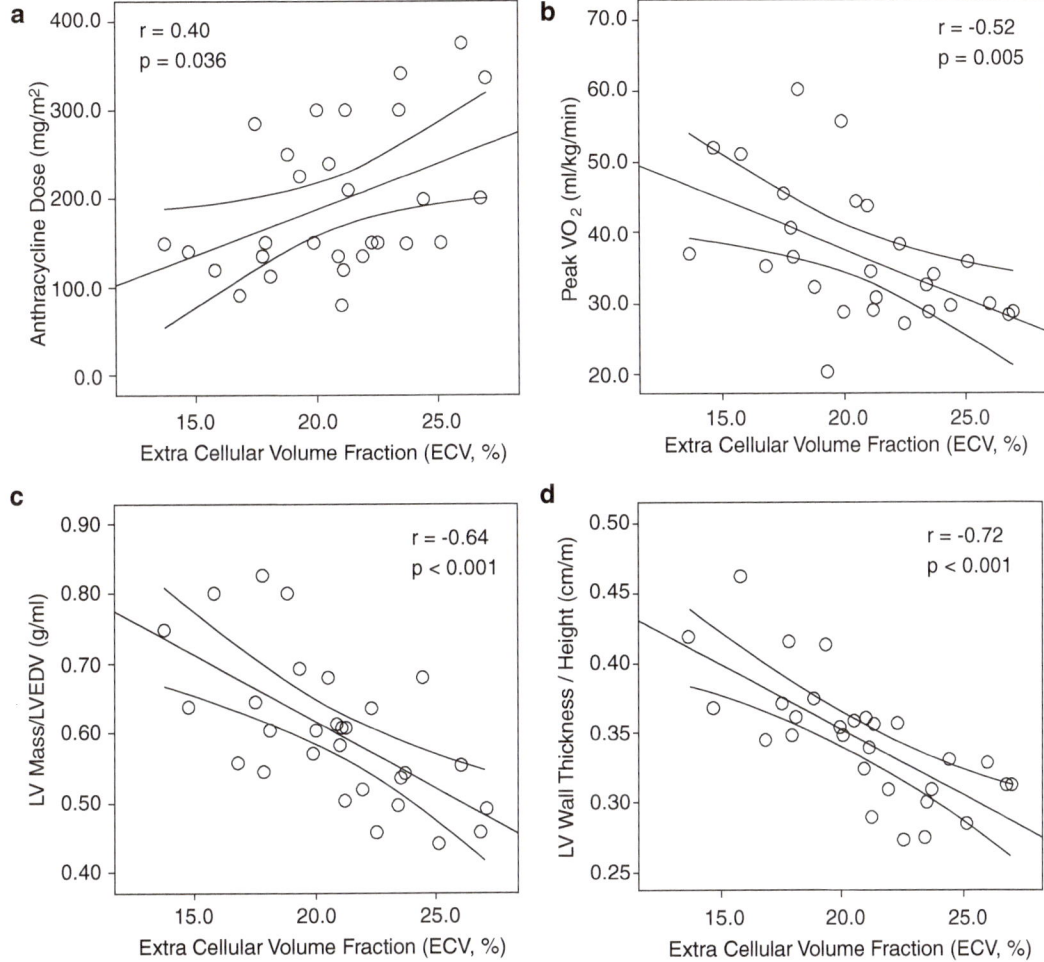

Fig. 3.8 Elevations in ECV of pediatric survivors treated with anthracycline chemotherapy correlates with markers of cardiovascular dysfunction and heart failure. Correlation of extracellular volume fraction (ECV) with (**a**) anthracycline dose, (**b**) peak VO2, (**c**) left ventricular mass/LVEDV and (**d**) LV wall thickness/height in 30 asymptomatic pediatric cancer survivors treated with anthracycline chemotherapy 7.6 ± 4.5 years prior to ECV imaging. Reprinted with permission under Open Access from [72]

New Challenges in T1 Mapping in Cardio-oncology

Challenges and limitations still remain in the application of T1 mapping to assess cardiomyopathy from cancer therapy. There is a growing concern in the use of gadolinium-based contrast agents, particularly in those who receive serial contrast exams [78–80]. This may limit the utility of contrast T1 and ECV mapping in this population for serial surveillance. Emerging non-contrast techniques and variants of T1 mapping, such as T1-rho mapping [81–83] and mag-netization transfer mapping, should be evaluated in this population and considered for use in those unable to receive gadolinium contrast for ECV and fibrosis quantification. Furthermore, there is now increasing evidence of both early myocardial fibrosis and acute injury in cancer patients; however, reliable discrimination of these disease entities continues to be difficult but presents opportunities for recovery as presented in Fig. 3.12 [10, 74, 84]. Delineation of the complex cardiovascular pathologies that occur after cancer treatment (Table 3.2) could be aided by T2 mapping or the use of biomarkers.

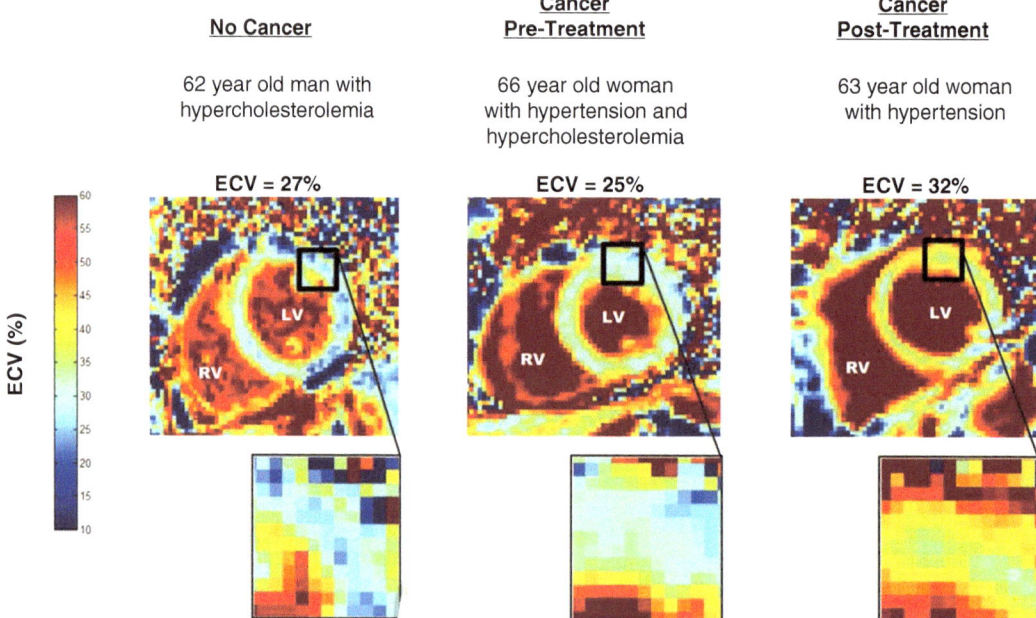

Fig. 3.9 Case examples of ECV maps demonstrating elevated ECV in a cancer survivor treated with anthracycline. Representative ECV maps from three participants of similar age and comorbidity burden either without cancer (left), newly diagnosed cancer yet to receive treatment (middle), and 2 years after cancer treatment (right) exhibiting diffuse increases in elevated extracellular volume of the cancer survivor. Reprinted with permission from [74]

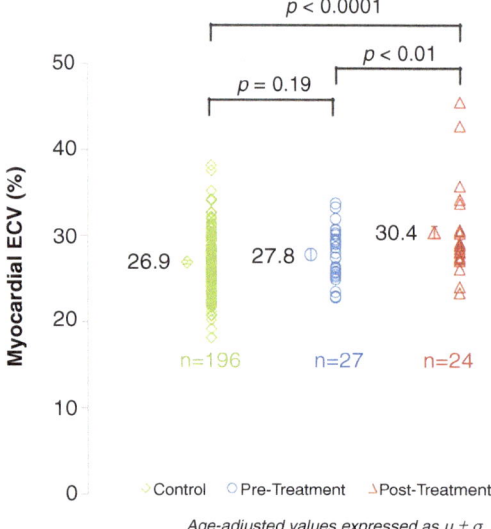

Fig. 3.10 Aggregate data of myocardial ECV demonstrating elevated ECV in cancer survivors. Myocardial extracellular volume (ECV) assessments of 2-year post-anthracycline cancer patients (right, red triangle) are elevated compared to newly diagnosed cancer patients yet to begin treatment (middle, blue circle) and cancer-free comparators from the Multi-Ethnic Study of Atherosclerosis (left, green diamond). ECV incrementally increases across each group (p < 0.0001). Reprinted with permission from [74]

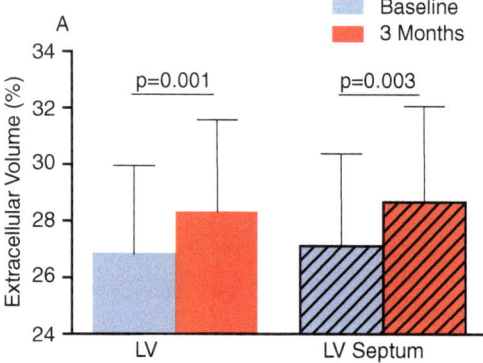

Fig. 3.11 Increases in myocardial fibrosis measured with CMR ECV may occur as early as 3 months after receipt of chemotherapy. Extracellular volume (ECV) analysis displaying the mean ± standard deviations before (blue) and 3 months after (red) initiation of chemotherapy. ECV was evaluated in the entire LV short axis (average of all accepted segments, solid bars) and in the LV septum (striped bars). Image courtesy Giselle C. Meléndez, MD (Wake Forest School of Medicine, Winston-Salem, North Carolina)

Table 3.3 CMR Protocol for assessment of cardiomyopathy and cancer treatment effects in cancer patients

Scan	Assessment
Localizers	Extra-cardiac abnormalities including metastases and aortic stenosis/enlargement
Long axis (LAX) cines(2, 3, 4 Chamber)	Myocardial contractility Wall motion abnormalities Global longitudinal strain
Short axis (SAX) cines	LV volumes and mass Wall motion abnormalities Circumferential strain
Native T1 mapping(3 SAX + 3 LAX views)	Inflammation Edema Fibrosis
T2 mapping(3 SAX + 3 LAX views)	Inflammation Edema
Tagging (3 SAX + 3 LAX views)	Global longitudinal strain Circumferential strain
If eligible, administer Gadolinium (Gd) contrast agent	
Post-Gd T1 mapping(3 SAX + 3 LAX views)	Fibrosis
TI scout	Inversion time determination
Late gadolinium enhancement(SAX stack + 3 LAX views)	Fibrosis Microvascular obstruction

This table demonstrates the scans in a suggested CMR protocol for the cardio-oncology patient. If possible, gadolinium contrasted scans provide additive value in describing the etiology of cardiovascular dysfunction

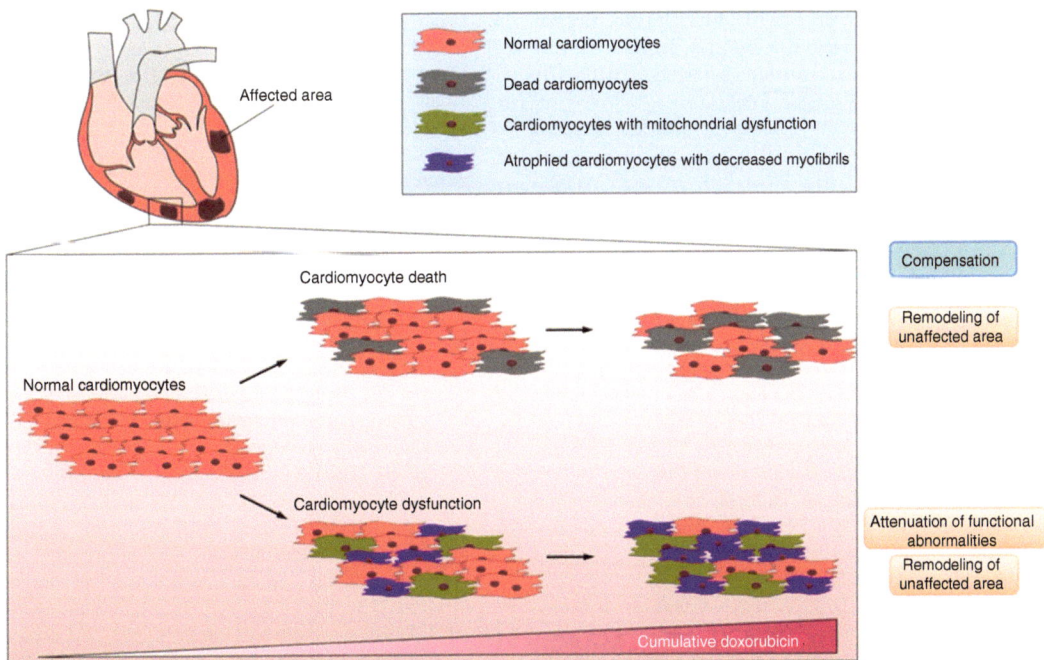

Fig. 3.12 Potential mechanisms for recovery from doxorubicin-induced cardiomyopathy. Cardiotoxicity is complex, multifactorial process that includes both irreversible cardiomyocyte death and potentially reversible dysfunction (e.g., mitochondrial defects, atrophy, and myofibrillar loss). Interventions aimed at attenuating dysfunction or compensating with the uninvolved myocardium may present opportunities for mitigating cardiotoxic effects in the myocardium. Reprinted with permission from [84]

Summary

To date, the vast majority of cardio-oncology research has focused on myocellular injury and LV dysfunction. Current surveillance strategies focused only on LVEF after symptoms may miss the onset of subclinical fibrosis and other early pathophysiologic manifestations, which require different therapy to prevent myocellular injury. Early work, utilizing T1 and ECV mapping in cardio-oncologic clinical studies, serves as a foundation for additional research to investigate the onset of myocardial fibrosis and its relation to cardiovascular mortality and exercise intolerance observed in cancer survivors. New clinical pathways are necessary to detect this early disease process to improve the cardiovascular health of cancer survivors.

References

1. Miller KD, Siegel RL, Lin CC, Mariotto AB, Kramer JL, Rowland JH, Stein KD, Alteri R, Jemal A. Cancer treatment and survivorship statistics, 2016. CA Cancer J Clin. 2016;66:271–89.
2. Siegel RL, Miller KD, Jemal A. Cancer statistics, 2016. CA Cancer J Clin. 2016;66:7–30.
3. Torre LA, Siegel RL, Ward EM, Jemal A. Global cancer incidence and mortality rates and trends—an update. Cancer Epidemiol Biomarkers Prev. 2016;25:16–27.
4. Berry GJ, Jorden M. Pathology of radiation and anthracycline cardiotoxicity. Pediatr Blood Cancer. 2005;44:630–7.
5. Grenier MA, Lipshultz SE. Epidemiology of anthracycline cardiotoxicity in children and adults. Semin Oncol. 1998;25:72–85.
6. Siegel R, Ma J, Zou Z, Jemal A. Cancer statistics, 2014. CA Cancer J Clin. 2014;64:9–29.
7. Okwuosa TM, Barac A. Burgeoning cardio-oncology programs challenges and opportunities for early career cardiologists/faculty directors. J Am Coll Cardiol. 2015;66:1193–6.
8. Hortobagyi GN. Drug therapy—treatment of breast cancer. N Engl J Med. 1998;339:974–84.
9. Lipshultz SE, Colan SD, Gelber RD, Perezatayde AR, Sallan SE, Sanders SP. Late cardiac effects of doxorubicin therapy for acute lymphoblastic-leukemia in childhood. N Engl J Med. 1991;324:808–15.
10. Meléndez GC, Hundley WG. Is myocardial fibrosis a new frontier for discovery in cardiotoxicity related to the administration of anthracyclines? Circ Cardiovasc Imaging. 2016;9(12).
11. Singal PK, Iliskovic N. Doxorubicin-induced cardiomyopathy. N Engl J Med. 1998;339:900–5.
12. Torti FM, Aston D, Lum BL, Kohler M, Williams R, Spaulding JT, Shortliffe L, Freiha FS. Weekly doxorubicin in endocrine refractory carcinoma of the prostate. J Clin Oncol. 1983;1:477–82.
13. Valdivieso M, Burgess MA, Ewer MS, Mackay B, Wallace S, Benjamin RS, Ali MK, Bodey GP, Freireich EJ. Increased therapeutic index of weekly doxorubicin in the therapy of non-small cell lung cancer—a prospective, randomized study. J Clin Oncol. 1984;2:207–14.
14. Mulrooney DA, Yeazel MW, Kawashima T, Mertens AC, Mitby P, Stovall M, Donaldson SS, Green DM, Sklar CA, Robison LL. Cardiac outcomes in a cohort of adult survivors of childhood and adolescent cancer: retrospective analysis of the Childhood Cancer Survivor Study cohort. BMJ. 2009;339:b4606.
15. Oeffinger KC, Mertens AC, Sklar CA, Kawashima T, Hudson MM, Meadows AT, Friedman DL, Marina N, Hobbie W, Kadan-Lottick NS, Schwartz CL, Leisenring W, Robison LL. Chronic health conditions in adult survivors of childhood cancer. N Engl J Med. 2006;355:1572–82.
16. Lipshultz SE, Alvarez JA, Scully RE. Anthracycline associated cardiotoxicity in survivors of childhood cancer. Heart. 2008;94:525–33.
17. Breast Cancer Facts & Figures 2011–2012. Atlanta: American Cancer Society, Inc.
18. Shankar SM, Marina N, Hudson MM, Hodgson DC, Adams MJ, Landier W, Bhatia S, Meeske K, Chen MH, Kinahan KE, Steinberger J, Rosenthal D. Monitoring for cardiovascular disease in survivors of childhood cancer: report from the Cardiovascular Disease Task Force of the Children's Oncology Group. Pediatrics. 2008;121:e387–96.
19. Patnaik JL, Byers T, Diguiseppi C, Dabelea D, Denberg TD. Cardiovascular disease competes with breast cancer as the leading cause of death for older females diagnosed with breast cancer: A retrospective cohort study. Breast Cancer Res. 2011;13:R64.
20. Sawyer DB, Peng X, Chen B, Pentassuglia L, Lim CC. Mechanisms of anthracycline cardiac injury: can we identify strategies for cardioprotection? Prog Cardiovasc Dis. 2010;53:105–13.
21. Zhu S-G, Kukreja RC, Das A, Chen Q, Lesnefsky EJ, Xi L. Dietary nitrate supplementation protects against doxorubicin-induced cardiomyopathy by improving mitochondrial function. J Am Coll Cardiol. 2011;57:2181–9.
22. An J, Li P, Li J, Dietz R, Donath S. ARC is a critical cardiomyocyte survival switch in doxorubicin cardiotoxicity. J Mol Med. 2009;87:401–10.
23. Childs AC, Phaneuf SL, Dirks AJ, Phillips T, Leeuwenburgh C. Doxorubicin treatment in vivo causes cytochrome C release and cardiomyocyte apoptosis, as well as increased mitochondrial efficiency, superoxide dismutase activity, and Bcl-2:Bax ratio. Cancer Res. 2002;62:4592–8.

24. Sorensen BS, Sinding J, Andersen AH, Alsner J, Jensen PB, Westergaard O. Mode of action of topoisomerase II-targeting agents at a specific DNA sequence: uncoupling the DNA binding, cleavage and religation events. J Mol Biol. 1992;228:778–86.

25. Kim Y, Ma AG, Kitta K, Fitch SN, Ikeda T, Ihara Y, Simon AR, Evans T, Suzuki YJ. Anthracycline-induced suppression of GATA-4 transcription factor: implication in the regulation of cardiac myocyte apoptosis. Mol Pharmacol. 2003;63:368–77.

26. Huang C, Zhang X, Ramil JM, Rikka S, Kim L, Lee Y, Gude NA, Thistlethwaite PA, Sussman MA, Gottlieb RA. Juvenile exposure to anthracyclines impairs cardiac progenitor cell function and vascularization resulting in greater susceptibility to stress-induced myocardial injury in adult mice. Circulation. 2010;121:675–83.

27. Cosper PF, Leinwand LA. Cancer causes cardiac atrophy and autophagy in a sexually dimorphic manner. Cancer Res. 2011;71:1710–20.

28. Zhao Y, Mclaughlin D, Robinson E, Harvey AP, Hookham MB, Shah AM, Mcdermott BJ, Grieve DJ. Nox2 NADPH oxidase promotes pathologic cardiac remodeling associated with Doxorubicin chemotherapy. Cancer Res. 2010;70:9287–97.

29. Peng X, Chen B, Lim CC, Sawyer DB. The cardiotoxicology of anthracycline chemotherapeutics: translating molecular mechanism into preventative medicine. Mol Interv. 2005;5:163–71.

30. Mewton N, Liu CY, Croisille P, Bluemke D, Lima JAC. Assessment of myocardial fibrosis with cardiovascular magnetic resonance. J Am Coll Cardiol. 2011;57:891–903.

31. Thavendiranathan P, Wintersperger BJ, Flamm SD, Marwick TH. Cardiac MRI in the assessment of cardiac injury and toxicity from cancer chemotherapy: a systematic review. Circ Cardiovasc Imaging. 2013b;6:1080–91.

32. Vasu S, Hundley WG. Understanding cardiovascular injury after treatment for cancer: an overview of current uses and future directions of cardiovascular magnetic resonance. J Cardiovasc Magn Reson. 2013;15:66–83.

33. Bovelli D, Plataniotis G, Roila F, Group, E. G. W. Cardiotoxicity of chemotherapeutic agents and radiotherapy-related heart disease: ESMO clinical practice guidelines. Ann Oncol. 2010;21:v277–82.

34. Fallah-Rad N, Walker JR, Wassef A, Lytwyn M, Bohonis S, Fang T, Tian G, Kirkpatrick ID, Singal PK, Krahn M. The utility of cardiac biomarkers, tissue velocity and strain imaging, and cardiac magnetic resonance imaging in predicting early left ventricular dysfunction in patients with human epidermal growth factor receptor II–positive breast cancer treated with adjuvant trastuzumab therapy. J Am Coll Cardiol. 2011;57:2263–70.

35. Johnson DB, Balko JM, Compton ML, Chalkias S, Gorham J, Xu Y, Hicks M, Puzanov I, Alexander MR, Bloomer TL. Fulminant myocarditis with combination immune checkpoint blockade. N Engl J Med. 2016;375:1749–55.

36. Ewer MS, Yeh ET. Cancer and the heart: PMPH-USA; 2013.

37. Plana JC, Galderisi M, Barac A, Ewer MS, Ky B, Scherrer-Crosbie M, Ganame J, Sebag IA, Agler DA, Badano LP, Banchs J, Cardinale D, Carver J, Cerqueira M, Decara JM, Edvardsen T, Flamm SD, Force T, Griffin BP, Jerusalem G, Liu JE, Magalhaes A, Marwick T, Sanchez LY, Sicari R, Villarraga HR, Lancellotti P. Expert consensus for multimodality imaging evaluation of adult patients during and after cancer therapy: a report from the American Society of Echocardiography and the European Association of Cardiovascular Imaging. J Am Soc Echocardiogr. 2014;27:911–39.

38. Bellenger N, Burgess M, Ray S, Lahiri A, Coats A, Cleland J, Pennell D. Comparison of left ventricular ejection fraction and volumes in heart failure by echocardiography, radionuclide ventriculography and cardiovascular magnetic resonance. Are they interchangeable? Eur Heart J. 2000;21:1387–96.

39. Cardinale D, Colombo A, Bacchiani G, Tedeschi I, Meroni CA, Veglia F, Civelli M, Lamantia G, Colombo N, Curigliano G, Fiorentini C, Cipolla CM. Early detection of anthracycline cardiotoxicity and improvement with heart failure therapy. Circulation. 2015;131:1981–8.

40. Hundley WG, Bluemke DA, Finn JP, Flamm SD, Fogel MA, Friedrich MG, Ho VB, Jerosch-Herold M, Kramer CM, Manning WJ, Patel M, Pohost GM, Stillman AE, White RD, Woodard PK. ACCF/ACR/AHA/NASCI/SCMR 2010 expert consensus document on cardiovascular magnetic resonance: a report of the American College of Cardiology Foundation Task Force on Expert Consensus Documents. Circulation. 2010;121:2462–508.

41. Raman SV, Shah M, Mccarthy B, Garcia A, Ferketich AK. Multi-detector row cardiac computed tomography accurately quantifies right and left ventricular size and function compared with cardiac magnetic resonance. Am Heart J. 2006;151:736–44.

42. Thavendiranathan P, Grant AD, Negishi T, Plana JC, Popovic ZB, Marwick TH. Reproducibility of echocardiographic techniques for sequential assessment of left ventricular ejection fraction and volumes: application to patients undergoing cancer chemotherapy. J Am Coll Cardiol. 2013a;61:77–84.

43. Walker J, Bhullar N, Fallah-Rad N, Lytwyn M, Golian M, Fang T, Summers AR, Singal PK, Barac I, Kirkpatrick ID, Jassal DS. Role of three-dimensional echocardiography in breast cancer: comparison to two-dimensional echocardiography, multiple-gated acquisition scans, and cardiac magnetic resonance imaging. J Clin Oncol. 2010;28:3429–36.

44. Alexander J, Dainiak N, Berger HJ, Goldman L, Johnstone D, Reduto L, Duffy T, Schwartz P, Gottschalk A, Zaret BL. Serial assessment of doxorubicin cardiotoxicity with quantitative radionuclide angiocardiography. N Engl J Med. 1979;300:278–83.

45. Schwartz RG, Mckenzie WB, Alexander J, Sager P, D'Souza A, Manatunga A, Schwartz PE, Berger

HJ, Setaro J, Surkin L, et al. Congestive heart failure and left ventricular dysfunction complicating doxorubicin therapy. Seven-year experience using serial radionuclide angiocardiography. Am J Med. 1987;82:1109–18.

46. Walker CM, Saldana DA, Gladish GW, Dicks DL, Kicska G, Mitsumori LM, Reddy GP. Cardiac complications of oncologic therapy. Radiographics. 2013;33:1801–15.

47. Ewer MS, Ali MK, Mackay B, Wallace S, Valdivieso M, Legha SS, Benjamin RS, Haynie TP. A comparison of cardiac biopsy grades and ejection fraction estimations in patients receiving Adriamycin. J Clin Oncol. 1984;2:112–7.

48. Gottdiener JS, Mathisen DJ, Borer JS, Bonow RO, Myers CE, Barr LH, Schwartz DE, Bacharach SL, Green MV, Rosenberg SA. Doxorubicin cardiotoxicity—assessment of late left-ventricular dysfunction by radionuclide cineangiography. Ann Intern Med. 1981;94:430–5.

49. Ky B, Putt M, Sawaya H, French B, Januzzi JL, Sebag IA, Plana JC, Cohen V, Banchs J, Carver JR. Early increases in multiple biomarkers predict subsequent cardiotoxicity in patients with breast cancer treated with doxorubicin, taxanes, and trastuzumab. J Am Coll Cardiol. 2014;63:809–16.

50. Stoodley PW, Richards DA, Hui R, Boyd A, Harnett PR, Meikle SR, Clarke J, Thomas L. Two-dimensional myocardial strain imaging detects changes in left ventricular systolic function immediately after anthracycline chemotherapy. Eur J Echocardiogr. 2011;12:945–52.

51. Sawaya H, Sebag IA, Plana JC, Januzzi JL, Ky B, Cohen V, Gosavi S, Carver JR, Wiegers SE, Martin RP, Picard MH, Gerszten RE, Halpern EF, Passeri J, Kuter I, Scherrer-Crosbie M. Early detection and prediction of cardiotoxicity in chemotherapy-treated patients. Am J Cardiol. 2011;107:1375–80.

52. Thavendiranathan P, Poulin F, Lim KD, Plana JC, Woo A, Marwick TH. Use of myocardial strain imaging by echocardiography for the early detection of cardiotoxicity in patients during and after cancer chemotherapy: a systematic review. J Am Coll Cardiol. 2014;63:2751–68.

53. Lange SA, Ebner B, Wess A, Kogel M, Gajda M, Hitschold T, Jung J. Echocardiography signs of early cardiac impairment in patients with breast cancer and trastuzumab therapy. Clin Res Cardiol. 2012;101:415–26.

54. Marchandise B, Schroeder E, Bosly A, Doyen C, Weynants P, Kremer R, Pouleur H. Early detection of doxorubicin cardiotoxicity: interest of Doppler echocardiographic analysis of left ventricular filling dynamics. Am Heart J. 1989;118:92–8.

55. Stoddard MF, Seeger J, Liddell NE, Hadley TJ, Sullivan DM, Kupersmith J. Prolongation of isovolumetric relaxation time as assessed by Doppler echocardiography predicts doxorubicin-induced systolic dysfunction in humans. J Am Coll Cardiol. 1992;20:62–9.

56. Tassan-Mangina S, Codorean D, Metivier M, Costa B, Himberlin C, Jouannaud C, Blaise AM, Elaerts J, Nazeyrollas P. Tissue Doppler imaging and conventional echocardiography after anthracycline treatment in adults: early and late alterations of left ventricular function during a prospective study. Eur J Echocardiogr. 2006;7:141–6.

57. Aletras AH, Ding SJ, Balaban RS, Wen H. DENSE: displacement encoding with stimulated echoes in cardiac functional MRI. J Magn Reson. 1999;137:247–52.

58. Osman NF, Kerwin WS, Mcveigh ER, Prince JL. Cardiac motion tracking using CINE harmonic phase (HARP) magnetic resonance imaging. Magn Reson Med. 1999;42:1048–60.

59. Drafts BC, Twomley KM, D'Agostino R Jr, Lawrence J, Avis N, Ellis LR, Thohan V, Jordan J, Melin SA, Torti FM, Little WC, Hamilton CA, Hundley WG. Low to moderate dose anthracycline-based chemotherapy is associated with early noninvasive imaging evidence of subclinical cardiovascular disease. JACC Cardiovasc Imaging. 2013;6:877–85.

60. Kongbundansuk S, Hundley WG. Noninvasive imaging of cardiovascular injury related to the treatment of cancer. JACC Cardiovasc Imaging. 2014;7:824–38.

61. Jordan JH, Sukpraphrute B, Meléndez GC, Jolly M-P, D'Agostino RB, Hundley WG. Early myocardial strain changes during potentially cardiotoxic chemotherapy may occur as a result of reductions in left ventricular end-diastolic volume. Circulation. 2017;135:2575–7.

62. Meléndez GC, Sukpraphrute B, D'Agostino RB, Jordan JH, Klepin HD, Ellis L, Lamar Z, Vasu S, Lesser G, Burke GL. Frequency of left ventricular end-diastolic volume–mediated declines in ejection fraction in patients receiving potentially cardiotoxic cancer treatment. Am J Cardiol. 2017;119:1637–42.

63. Devita VT, Hellman S, Rosenberg SA. Cancer, principles & practice of oncology. Philadelphia, PA: Lippincott Williams & Wilkins; 2005.

64. Ferrans VJ. Overview of cardiac pathology in relation to anthracycline cardiotoxicity. Cancer Treat Rep. 1978;62:955–61.

65. Olson HM, Young DM, Prieur DJ, Leroy AF, Reagan RL. Electrolyte and morphologic alterations of myocardium in adriamycin-treated rabbits. Am J Pathol. 1974;77:439–54.

66. Cottin Y, Ribuot C, Maupoil V, Godin D, Arnould L, Brunotte F, Rochette L. Early incidence of adriamycin treatment on cardiac parameters in the rat. Can J Physiol Pharmacol. 1994;72:140–5.

67. Thompson RC, Canby RC, Lojeski EW, Ratner AV, Fallon JT, Pohost GM. Adriamycin cardiotoxicity and proton nuclear-magnetic-resonance relaxation properties. Am Heart J. 1987;113:1444–9.

68. Wassmuth R, Lentzsch S, Erdbruegger U, Schulz-Menger J, Doerken B, Dietz R, Friedrich MG. Subclinical cardiotoxic effects of anthracyclines as assessed by magnetic resonance imaging—a pilot study. Am Heart J. 2001;141:1007–13.

69. Lightfoot JC, D'Agostino RB, Hamilton CA, Jordan J, Torti FM, Kock ND, Jordan J, Workman S, Hundley WG. Novel approach to early detection of doxorubicin cardiotoxicity by gadolinium-enhanced cardiovascular magnetic resonance imaging. Circ Cardiovasc Imaging. 2010;3(5):550–8. https://doi.org/10.1161/CIRCIMAGING.109.918540.

70. Jordan JH, D'Agostino RB, Hamilton CA, Vasu S, Hall ME, Kitzman DW, Thohan V, Lawrence JA, Ellis LR, Lash TL. Longitudinal assessment of concurrent changes in left ventricular ejection fraction and left ventricular myocardial tissue characteristics after administration of cardiotoxic chemotherapies using T1-weighted and T2-weighted cardiovascular magnetic resonance. Circ Cardiovasc Imaging. 2014;7:872–9.

71. Neilan TG, Coelho OR, Shah RV, Feng JZH, Pena-Herrera D, Mandry D, Pierre-Mongeon F, Heydari B, Francis SA, Moslehi J, Kwong RY, Jerosch-Herold M. Myocardial extracellular volume by cardiac magnetic resonance imaging in patients treated with anthracycline-based chemotherapy. Am J Cardiol. 2013;111:717–22.

72. Tham EB, Haykowsky MJ, Chow K, Spavor M, Kaneko S, Khoo NS, Pagano JJ, Mackie AS, Thompson RB. Diffuse myocardial fibrosis by T1-mapping in children with subclinical anthracycline cardiotoxicity: Relationship to exercise capacity, cumulative dose and remodeling. J Cardiovasc Magn Reson. 2013;15:48.

73. Toro-Salazar OH, Gillan E, O'Loughlin M, Burke GS, Ferranti J, Stainsby J, Liang B, Mazur W, Raman S, Hor K. Occult cardiotoxicity in childhood cancer survivors exposed to anthracycline therapy. Circ Cardiovasc Imaging. 2013;6(6):873–80.

74. Jordan JH, Vasu S, Morgan TM, D'Agostino RB Jr, Meléndez GC, Hamilton CA, Arai AE, Liu S, Liu CY, Lima JAC, Bluemke DA, Burke GL, Hundley WG. Anthracycline-associated T1 mapping characteristics are elevated independent of the presence of cardiovascular comorbidities in cancer survivors. Circ Cardiovasc Imaging. 2016;9(8). https://doi.org/10.1161/CIRCIMAGING.115.004325.

75. Meléndez GC, Jordan JH, D'Agostino RB Jr, Vasu S, Hamilton CA, Hundley WG. Progressive three-month increase in left ventricular myocardial extracellular volume fraction after receipt of anthracycline based

chemotherapy. JACC Cardiovasc Imaging. 2016. https://doi.org/10.1016/j.jcmg.2016.06.006.

76. Farhad H, Staziaki PV, Addison D, Coelho-Filho OR, Shah RV, Mitchell RN, Szilveszter B, Abbasi SA, Kwong RY, Scherrer-Crosbie M. Characterization of the changes in cardiac structure and function in mice treated with anthracyclines using serial cardiac magnetic resonance imaging. Circ Cardiovasc Imaging. 2016;9:e003584.

77. Shelburne N, Adhikari B, Brell J, Davis M, Desvigne-Nickens P, Freedman A, Minasian L, Force T, Remick SC. Cancer treatment-related cardiotoxicity: current state of knowledge and future research priorities. J Natl Cancer Inst. 2014;106(9).

78. Mcdonald RJ, Mcdonald JS, Kallmes DF, Jentoft ME, Murray DL, Thielen KR, Williamson EE, Eckel LJ. Intracranial gadolinium deposition after contrast-enhanced MR imaging. Radiology. 2015;275:772–82.

79. Montagne A, Toga AW, Zlokovic BV. Blood-brain barrier permeability and gadolinium: benefits and potential pitfalls in research. JAMA Neurol. 2016;73:13–4.

80. Murata N, Gonzalez-Cuyar LF, Murata K, Fligner C, Dills R, Hippe D, Maravilla KR. Macrocyclic and other non–group 1 gadolinium contrast agents deposit low levels of gadolinium in brain and bone tissue: preliminary results from 9 patients with normal renal function. Investig Radiol. 2016;51:447–53.

81. Berisha S, Han J, Shahid M, Han Y, Witschey WR. Measurement of myocardial T1ρ with a motion corrected, parametric mapping sequence in humans. PLoS One. 2016;11:e0151144.

82. Stromp TA, Leung SW, Andres KN, Jing L, Fornwalt BK, Charnigo RJ, Sorrell VL, Vandsburger MH. Gadolinium free cardiovascular magnetic resonance with 2-point Cine balanced steady state free precession. J Cardiovasc Magn Reson. 2015;17:90.

83. Van Oorschot JW, Visser F, Eikendal AL, Vonken E-JP, Luijten PR, Chamuleau SA, Leiner T, Zwanenburg JJ. Single breath-hold T1ρ-mapping of the heart for endogenous assessment of myocardial fibrosis. Investig Radiol. 2016;51:505–12.

84. Moslehi J, Amgalan D, Kitsis RN. Grounding cardio-oncology in basic and clinical science. Circulation. 2017;136:3–5.

Comparison of T1 Mapping by Cardiac MRI to Non-cardiac MRI Methods to Evaluate Cardiac Fibrosis

4

Róisín B. Morgan, Michael Jerosch-Herold, and Raymond Y. Kwong

Introduction

Myocardial fibrosis is a pathological process involving extracellular matrix (ECM) remodeling.

In practical terms, the two basic types of fibrosis are focal and diffuse. Focal fibrosis is defined as scar (e.g., myocardial infarction) or focal patches of scar interspersed within the normal myocardium, as is the case in many cardiomyopathies. Conversely, the presence of diffuse, reactive fibrosis is increasingly recognized in a variety of conditions, even in the absence of myocardial ischemia. The structure and composition of the myocardial extracellular matrix (ECM) ensure the harmonic structure and function of the heart and mediate cell to cell and cell to ECM molecular signaling and interactions [1]. In myocardial disease, increased ECM deposition is a crucial compensatory and repair process. Replacement fibrosis, a process that typically occurs after the loss of cardiomyocytes post–

myocardial infarction (MI), contributes to maintaining the macroanatomy of the heart. On the other hand, reactive fibrosis occurs in response to cardiac stress and is seen in most cardiac diseases with pressure [2] and volume overload [3], underlying cardiomyopathy such as HCM [4], ARVC [5] or DCM [6], and in areas of post-MI remodeling in the noninfarcted area [7].

Regardless of the etiology, fibrosis causes increased myocardial stiffness thus promoting cardiac dysfunction. Clinically, these patients present with symptoms of cardiac failure although in many cases this is a subclinical disease and may present at a later stage. As discussed in this chapter, imaging techniques such as echocardiography, cardiac magnetic resonance (CMR), multidetector cardiac computed tomography (MDCT) and nuclear imaging have been proven to detect early features of systolic and diastolic left ventricular (LV) dysfunction and impaired contractile reserve. The evolving field of CMR and molecular techniques may shortly lead to the further identification of diffuse reactive fibrosis. The goal of such new modalities is to promote and enable targeted therapy to be instituted earlier, thus, leading to prevention of disease progression and fibrosis accumulation long term.

Traditionally, endomyocardial biopsy has been the method utilized for quantification of myocardial interstitial collagen content. However, imaging techniques and serum collagen biomarkers may be used as surrogate markers of

R. B. Morgan · R. Y. Kwong (✉)
Non-invasive Cardiovascular Imaging, Cardiovascular Division, Department of Medicine, Brigham and Women's Hospital, Harvard Medical School, Boston, MA, USA
e-mail: rmorgan@mmc.org; rykwong@partners.org

M. Jerosch-Herold
Department of Radiology, Brigham and Women's Hospital, Harvard Medical School, Boston, MA, USA
e-mail: mjerosch-herold@bwh.harvard.edu

© Springer International Publishing AG, part of Springer Nature 2018
P. C. Yang (ed.), *T1-Mapping in Myocardial Disease*, https://doi.org/10.1007/978-3-319-91110-6_4

myocardial fibrosis [8]. These imaging methods may be divided into methods to visualize fibrosis (CMR, MDCT, and nuclear imaging) and techniques to assess subtle subclinical LV systolic and diastolic dysfunction (predominantly echocardiographic). These methods are discussed in detail below.

Cardiac MRI (CMR)

In CMR imaging, the signal intensity of the pixel is based on the relaxation of hydrogen nuclei protons in the static magnetic field, the strength of which is measured in Tesla (T), and typically 1.5 or 3.0T for cardiac imaging. The relaxation of the hydrogen nucleus proton is characterized by two very distinct MR relaxation parameters. First, the T1 or spin-lattice relaxation time corresponds to a specific time constant when the 1H nuclear magnetization has recovered to roughly 63% of its equilibrium value after magnetization inversion. Secondly, the transverse relaxation time (T2) or spin-spin relaxation time corresponds to the specific time when the 1H transverse magnetization created by a radio-frequency (RF) pulse excitation drops to roughly 37% of its initial value right after the RF pulse [9]. Both of these time constants depend on the molecular environment of the water molecules in the tissue and thus they characterize each tissue specifically. Times vary significantly from one type of tissue to another, but also can vary within the same tissue depending on its pathophysiological status (e.g. inflammation, edema, fibrosis).

Late gadolinium enhancement cardiac MRI (LGE-CMR) has become the clinical reference standard for determining the presence and extent of myocardial infarction in ischemic heart disease. For nonischemic cardiomyopathy, it has become an effective tool providing an accurate, non-invasive detection of focal myocardial fibrosis with both diagnostic and prognosis values. It has been extensively validated against histopathological examination in nonischemic conditions [10, 11] and ischemic heart disease [12]. After injection of intravenous gadolinium contrast (Gd), distinct enhancement patterns occur in different myocardial disorders, all characterized by tissue disarray, fibrosis, and inflammation [13–17]. Regardless of the etiology, myocyte injury typically leads to increased myocardial collagen content and a marked reduction of cardiomyocyte volume [18]. Gd-based contrast agents permeate the extra-cellular space, leading to enhancement in regions of focal myocardial necrosis. The physiological basis of the LGE of myocardial fibrosis is based on the combination of an increased volume of distribution for the contrast agent and a prolonged wash-out related to the decreased capillary density within the myocardial fibrotic tissue [12, 19]. In CMR, the discrimination between scarred/fibrotic myocardium and normal myocardium relies on contrast concentration differences in addition to the chosen setting of the inversion-recovery sequence parameters (TI-time). These parameters are set to "null" the normal myocardial signal that appears dark in the final image relative to the bright signal of the scarred/fibrotic myocardium as shown in Fig. 4.1 [9].

Although LGE-CMR allows a very sensitive and reproducible qualitative assessment of myocardial replacement fibrosis, it is limited to cases where focal necrosis produces a localized loss of cardiomyocytes, that can be contrasted against other regions in the heart that remain viable. A diffuse loss of cardiomyocytes and concurrent expansion of the extra-cellular matrix can be difficult to visualize and quantify with LGE imaging, as it resembles more of a binary diagnostic test, rather than a method that can detect the build-up of fibrosis as a continuum. As a result, in recent years T1 and T2 mapping techniques have been developed by the CMR community to quantify myocardial fibrosis accurately. Recent technical improvements in acquisition sequences have enabled us to perform myocardial T1mapping with high spatial resolution by using both 1.5 and 3T magnetic resonance imaging scanners within a single breath hold [20, 21]. Compared with LGE imaging, T1 mapping by CMR before and after contrast administration provides a continuous measure of extra-cellular volume (ECV) expansion that correlates in my cardiac conditions closely with the build-up of

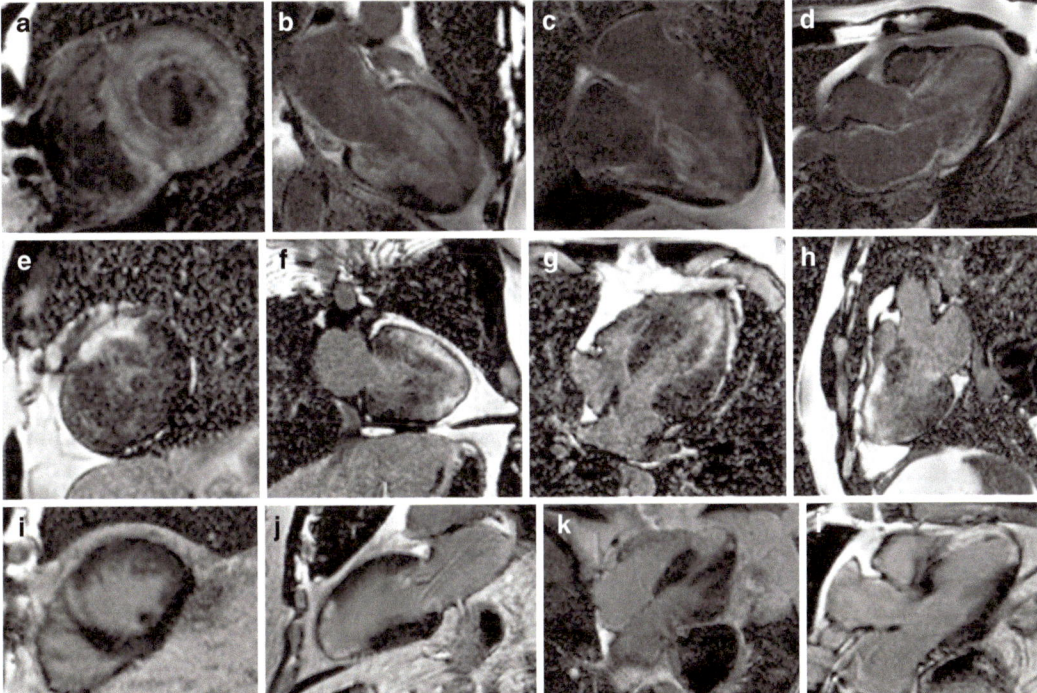

Fig. 4.1 LGE-CMR images from patients with myocardial fibrosis caused by cardiac amyloidosis (**a–d**), hypertrophic cardiomyopathy (**e–h**) and ischemic cardiomyopathy with evidence of prior subendocardial infarction in the distribution of the distal LAD (**i–l**). Gadolinium contrast media accumulates in the abnormal fibrotic myocardium and appears bright in contrast to the normal myocardium (dark). The distribution and extent of LGE in these examples are classic for the associated condition

interstitial fibrosis. It thus allows quantification of ECV on a standardized scale of each myocardial voxel to characterize myocardial tissue [9]. The myocardial native T1 (i.e. measured without giving any contrast agent) can by itself also provide an indication of tissue pathology, but in the case of diffuse fibrosis the origin of changes in native T1 can encompass a range of conditions such as edema, and also the build of connective tissue.

In practice, by reconstructing a sequence of images corresponding to various times after an magnetization inversion (TI), T1 maps can be generated in which each pixel intensity value represents the T1 relaxation time (e.g., in ms). A key requirement is that all images are acquired in the same of the cardiac cycle, so that the inversion recovery can be tracked for single pixels. For this purpose, Messroghli et al. [20] introduced the Modified Look-Locker Inversion-recovery

(MOLLI) sequence, which has become a standard in CMR T1 mapping. More recently, a short MOLLI (modified Look-Locker inversion recovery) sequence has been described, which approximately halved the required breath hold duration and the number of required heartbeats decreased from 17 to 9 [21], but requires more complex processing to generate T1 maps. From a clinical perspective, shMOLLI has enabled significant reduction of the duration of the scan and the quality of the T1 maps is arguably improved due to shorter breath hold time and reduced residual motion.

Areas of diffuse myocardial fibrosis have greater T1 values than normal tissue before intravenous Gd-based contrast media (Gd) is given. Post-Gd administration, T1 value is lower than normal in diffuse myocardial fibrosis. The reason for this lies in the fact that the expanded extracellular space in diffuse fibrosis accumulates more

Gd-based contrast than the healthy tissue with compact myocytes. A reduction in T1 value is not specific for diffuse myocardial fibrosis; however, T1 reduction may also occur with cardiomyopathies where the extracellular space is expanded such as in amyloid depositions [22].

A number of validation studies have been carried out comparing histology to T1 mapping and ECV values. That being said, Iles et al. [23] examined a symptomatic heterogeneous heart failure population using post-contrast MOLLI. They compared post-transplant myocardial biopsies with T1 values and demonstrated an inverse correlation between T1 values with percentage fibrosis. They also found a reduction in T1 with worsening diastolic function. Sibley et al. used a post-contrast Look-Locker technique and also demonstrated an inverse correlation between T1 time and histological fibrosis on myocardial biopsy in patients with a broad range of cardiomyopathies [24]. Studies that are based on the use of post-contrast T1, rather than derivation of ECV, for the detection of diffuse fibrosis, require careful standardization of the time between contrast-injection and T1 mapping, to eliminate the potential confounding variable of contrast clearance times. Furthermore, the post-contrast T1 will also depend on the rate of renal clearance of the contrast agent, introducing the patients' renal function as additional confounder. ECV, which is calculated as the change of the myocardial T1 rate constants (inverse of the measured myocardial T1) between pre- and post-contrast states, normalized by the change of the blood T1 rate constants (inverse of the measured blood T1), is largely independent of the rate of contrast clearance. Also, ECV values are also independent of scanner field strength since this measurement is a ratio of the changes in myocardial-blood rate constants, which is in contrast to T1 values that increase with field strength both for native- and post-contrast T1 measurements. Robustness of ECV derivation is also enhanced by capturing the myocardial and blood wash-in and wash-out dynamics during the 15–30 min period after Gd injection by acquiring multiple post-contrast T1 map in addition to the pre-contrast T1 map. Table 4.1 explores the various studies to date, investigating the use of T1 map in various cardiac conditions associated with myocardial fibrosis.

In practice, myocardial T1 mapping is technically demanding and standardization of the methodology is required. The CMR community has made a concerted effort at standardization [37]; however, in the coming years, the routine use of T1 map for clinical evaluation of myocardial fibrosis will become more user-friendly and less time-consuming for routine clinical practice.

Novel CMR Approaches

Concerns about the administration of Gd-bound contrast agents (GBCA) to patients with poor renal function have provided a strong impetus for developing CMR methods that do not rely on GBCA for the detection of diffuse fibrosis. With the standard imaging techniques, generally the signal from 1H nuclei in connective tissue components such as collagen is not detected due to the very short T2 constants for collagen 1H nuclei that are approximately 1 ms. Standard T1-mapping techniques such as MOLLI [38] do not detect or detect poorly the signal components from 1H nuclei in connective tissue. A direct detection of the 1H signal from connective tissue components such as collagen can be achieved with imaging sequences that use ultra-short echo times (UTE) on the order of a fraction of a millisecond. UTE imaging is increasingly seen as a promising approach for the detection of diffuse fibrosis by measuring the fraction of 1H signal that comes from connective tissue relative to the 1H signal from mobile 1H nuclei. Initial studies have demonstrated encouraging feasibility of this approach for detecting diffuse fibrosis [39]. The 1H signal from collagen is shifted relatively to the 1H from the mobile 1H nuclei by −3.2 ppm. The decay of the 1H signal from myocardial tissue as a function of the echo-time, therefore, can be described as a bi-exponential decay where the relatively quick decaying collagen component oscillates as a function of the 3.2 ppm 1H frequency shift for the collagen component. Using this type of model for the myocardial signal

Table 4.1 Data supporting the use of T1 mapping in the evaluation of myocardial fibrosis and the conditions studied

Author and date	Disease	Technique	Conclusion
Messroghli [25] 2003	Acute Myocardial Infarction	Look-Locker	In acute MI patients post-contrast T1 values were significantly lower than normal myocardium T1 values
Maceira [26] 2005	Amyloidosis	Look locker	Subepicardial post-contrast T1 values were significantly reduced in cardiac amyloidosis patients compared with controls
Messroghli [27] 2007	Myocardial infarction, acute or chronic	MOLLI	In acute and chronic myocardial infarction, pre-contrast T1 values were higher than T1 values in remote myocardium
Iles [23] 2008	Heart failure	VAST	Post-contrast myocardial T1 times correlated histologically with fibrosis and were shorter in heart failure subjects than controls (p 0.0001) [23]. The post-contrast myocardial T1 time reduced as diastolic function worsened
Broberg [28] 2010	Adult congenital heart disease	Look-Locker	Patients with ACHD have diffuse, extracellular matrix remodeling similar to patients with acquired heart failure as measured by T1 mapping
Flett [29] 2010	Aortic stenosis. HCM	Look-Locker	A high correlation was seen between T1 mapping with equilibrium contrast CMR and histologic fibrosis in aortic stenosis and HCM
Gai [30] 2011	Diabetes mellitus	Look-Locker	A significant difference was noted in post-contrast T1 values between those at low risk of diabetes compared with those at high risk
Bauner [31] 2012	Chronic MI	MOLLI	A significant difference was noted in post-contrast T1 values in chronic myocardial infarct regions compared to healthy myocardium
Turkbey [32] 2012	Myotonic Dystrophy	Look locker	Postcontrast myocardial T1 time was shorter in myotonic dystrophy patients compared to controls, likely reflecting the presence of diffuse myocardial fibrosis
Dass [33] 2012	HCM/DCM	ShMOLLI	HCM/DCM patients had higher pre-contrast T1 times than controls
Fontana [34] 2012	HCM, AS, amyloid	ShMOLLI	ECV quantification using single breath-hold ShMOLLI T1 mapping can measure ECV by EQ-CMR across a spectrum of interstitial expansion
Rao [35] 2013	Diabetes	Look locker	The myocardial ECV in this diabetic population was elevated compared with published values of ECV in healthy subjects and with the mean ECV of 0.27 ± 0.03 (p < 0.0001) obtained in healthy, normotensive volunteers
Ellims [36] 2014	Post-cardiac transplant	VAST	Diffuse myocardial fibrosis (as assessed by post-contrast myocardial T1 time), correlates with invasively-demonstrated LV stiffness in cardiac transplant patients
Ntusi 2015	Rheumatoid Arthritis	ShMOLLI	Focal fibrosis (LGE) was found in 46% of RA patients compared with none of the controls. Larger areas of focal myocardial edema were seen in patients with RA. They also had higher native T1 values, larger areas of involvement as indicated by native T1 > 990 ms and expansion of ECV compared with controls

decay as a function of TE, one can show that the collagen signal fraction changes linearly with collagen concentration [40], suggesting feasibility in fibrosis quantitation.

Another approach with the same goal of quantifying the connective tissue fraction in the myocardium is based on a technique termed chemical-exchange saturation transfer (CEST) imaging. The endogenous CEST between macromolecules in fibrotic scar tissue and surrounding water has been investigated in a murine model of myocardial infarction (MI). CEST contrast is generated through frequency-selective RF saturation to exchange the magnetization between scar tissue and surrounding water in normal myocardium, followed by image-acquisition. The signal read-out during the image-acquisition is thereby encoded by the molecular signature of the target tissue of interest (e.g. fibrotic tissue). A recent study [41] has shown the feasibility of detecting scar tissue though it remains uncertain whether the diffuse interstitial fibrosis, a more challenging target than infarct scar, can be quantified with this technique.

Another approach aimed at the direct detection of scar and fibrosis is based on the use of targeted contrast agents, specifically the use of collagen-binding contrast agents. In this type of contrast agents, the wash-out time constants in regions of post-infarction scar become significantly longer, compared to a Gd-based contrast agent without binding affinity for collagen or other myocardial scar components [42]. To-date it remains unclear if such collagen-binding contrast agents are also suitable for the detection of diffuse interstitial fibrosis. The approach for detecting diffuse interstitial fibrosis with a collagen-binding contrast agent is likely to involve T1-mapping to quantify collagen-bound fraction of contrast.

Nuclear Imaging

Molecular imaging techniques for detecting diffuse myocardial fibrosis using SPECT or PET imaging are predominantly research-based tools with great potential for future clinical use [1, 7, 43]. Ischemic fibrosis, however, may be readily detected, using myocardial perfusion techniques, which are currently in routine clinical practice.

Radionuclide imaging techniques are frequently used in the evaluation of patients with known or suspected CAD. These techniques use radiolabeled drugs or radiopharmaceuticals which are injected intravenously and trapped in myocardial tissue. Radioactivity within the heart decays by emitting gamma rays. The interaction between these gamma rays and the detectors in specialized scanners—single photon emission computed tomography (SPECT) and positron emission tomography (PET)—creates a scintillation event, which can be captured by digital recording equipment to create an image of the heart. Electrocardiogram (ECG)-triggered gated rest and stress images are acquired after intravenous injection of the radiopharmaceutical and used to define the extent and severity of myocardial ischemia and scar as well as regional and global cardiac function and remodeling. In SPECT imaging, technetium-99m (99mTc)-labeled tracers are frequently used because they generate the best image quality and the lowest radiation dose to the patient. After intravenous injection, these tracers become trapped intracellularly in mitochondria and show minimal change over time (Figs. 4.2 and 4.3).

PET myocardial perfusion imaging (MPI) is an alternative to SPECT and is associated with improved diagnostic accuracy and lower radiation dose to the patient. To evaluate myocardial viability in post-MI patients, myocardial perfusion imaging with SPECT or PET usually is combined with metabolic imaging—specifically, 18F-fluorodeoxyglucose (FDG) PET. The presence of a reversible myocardial perfusion defect is indicative of ischemia whereas a fixed perfusion defect generally reflects scarred myocardium (area of fibrosis) from previous infarction. 18F-FDG is used to assess regional myocardial glucose utilization and compared to perfusion

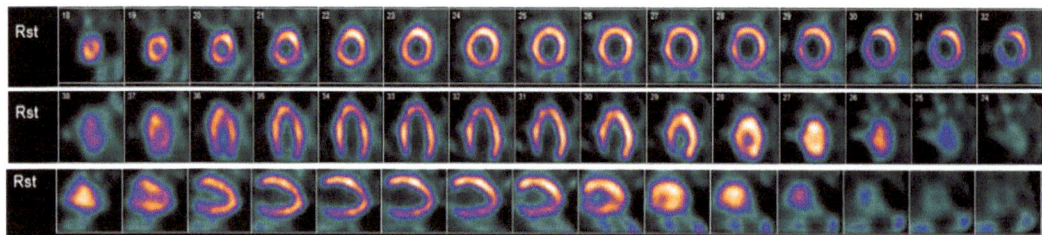

Fig. 4.2 Rest myocardial perfusion images in a normal patient with normal myocardial uptake of sestamibi seen in short axis, vertical long axis and horizontal long axis images (top, middle and bottom rows respectively)

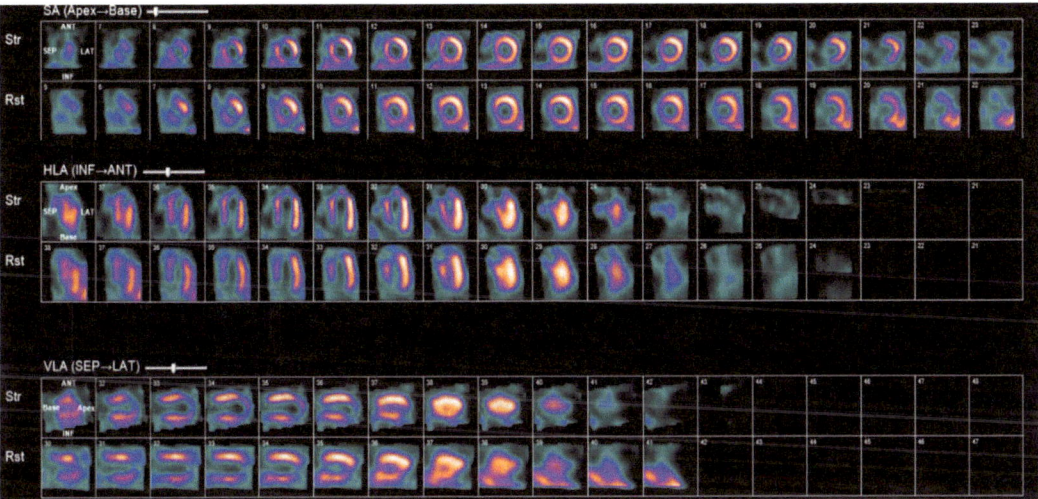

Fig. 4.3 Stress (top row) and rest perfusion (bottom row) images in a patient with a medium to large region of myocardial fibrosis (scar) in the distribution of the mid left anterior descending (LAD) artery, with minimal ischemia

images to define metabolic abnormalities associated with infarction and hibernation. Myocardial regions showing reduced perfusion and increased FDG uptake at rest (so-called *perfusion-FDG mismatch*) identify areas of viable but hibernating myocardium, whereas regions showing reduced perfusion and FDG uptake at rest (so-called *perfusion-FDG match*) are consistent with myocardial scar or fibrosis.

Using $H2^{15}O$ and $C^{15}O$ tracers, PET can assess the perfusable tissue index (PTI), i.e. the fraction of the myocardium that is perfusable by water [44]. As fibrotic myocardium is unable to exchange water rapidly, a reduction in this variable may correlate with fibrosis. PTI, reduced in patients with advanced dilated cardiomyopathy [45], correlates with reduced contractile function [46] and is also present in areas of focal fibrosis following MI [47]. However, its use has not been validated in a histological comparison study. Technetium-99m-labelled Cy5.5-RGD injection followed by PET imaging [48] has been shown in animal models as a tracer that binds to myofibroblast cells and correlates with new collagen deposition in an experimental model of myocardial infarction [7]. These techniques are not in routine clinical use, and although they have shown promising results, currently they are not applicable to patients in the current era.

Hypertrophic cardiomyopathy patients may show abnormalities and replacement fibrosis on myocardial SPECT and positron emission tomography (PET) indicative of underlying abnormalities of oxidative metabolism, which may precede myocardial perfusion abnormalities and replacement fibrosis [49]. Impaired metabolism has been noted in up to 73% of segments when radiotracers such as FDG, C-acetate or 123I-BIMPP were used; these observations suggest that the impairment of long-chain fatty acid metabolism may precede other metabolic abnormalities in HCM patients [50]. Another study examining myocardial fibrosis in HCM patients who underwent LGE-CMR, Tc99m-MIBI SPECT, and I23-BIMPP SPECT [51] showed that segments with a larger extent of replacement fibrosis on LGE-CMR had more abnormalities in perfusion and metabolism on SPECT.

Echocardiography

Backscatter

The reflectivity of tissue to ultrasound is a noninvasive measure of myocardial tissue characterization and collagen deposition that has been used for multiple decades [52]. Qualitative M-mode and 2D echo imaging techniques have been widely used for scar detection and wall motion assessment in ischemic fibrosis. In addition to these methods, backscatter techniques were developed in the 1980s to quantify myocardial tissue changes characteristic of fibrosis in conditions such as HCM and hypertension [53]. This quantitative echocardiographic estimation of fibrosis was predominantly performed via ultrasonic video densitometric and texture analysis [43]. The relationship between backscatter and histologically quantitated collagen has been confirmed in the literature [54]. Noninvasively, amplitudes of integrated backscatter have also been correlated with elevated pro-collagen concentration [55].

Two myocardial backscatter parameters have been established for use: (1) magnitude of cyclic variation in integrated backscatter, which is a marker of regional function, and although abnormal in conditions of diffuse fibrosis, this parameter has been largely replaced by myocardial strain, and (2) calibrated integrated backscatter. A greater calibrated integrated backscatter is indicative of larger fibrosis [43]. This technique has been used to establish a transmural trend of fibrosis in non-transmural infarction and hence could potentially be employed to assess fibrotic gradients in conditions, such as diabetic heart disease or Duchenne muscular dystrophy with predominantly endocardial or epicardial fibrosis, respectively [56, 57]. Elevated backscatter also occurs with systemic sclerosis although predominantly in the diffuse rather than the limited subgroup [58].

Tissue Doppler Imaging (TDI)

Doppler echocardiography relies on the detection of the shift in frequency of ultrasound signals reflected from moving objects. Conventional Doppler techniques evaluate the velocity of blood flow by measuring high frequency, low amplitude signals from small, fast-moving blood cells [59]. In Tissue Doppler imaging (TDI), these principals are used to quantify the high amplitude, low-velocity signals of myocardial tissue motion. This in turn serves as a measure of myocardial function, typically reduced in the fibrotic heart.

Pulsed wave TDI is used to measure peak myocardial velocities and performs well at the measurement of long-axis ventricular motion, mostly because the longitudinally oriented endocardial fibers are most parallel to the ultrasound beam in apical views of the heart.

Reduction of longitudinal function appears to be one of the most sensitive markers of subclinical heart disease in many conditions associated with fibrosis, including diabetes and hypertension [43]. The impairment of longitudinal function reflects the principal initial involvement of subendocardial fibers, followed by compensation by mid-wall fibers and subsequent improvement in radial contractility to maintain overall cardiac function [57].

Because the apex remains relatively stationary throughout the cardiac cycle, mitral annular motion is a good surrogate marker of overall longitudinal left ventricular contraction and relaxation [60]. Systolic myocardial velocity (Sa), measured at the lateral mitral annulus is a measure of longitudinal systolic function and has been correlated with measurements of LV ejection fraction (EF) [61]. When carrying out an assessment of left ventricular diastolic function, transmitral velocities are directly related to left atrial pressure (preload) and independently related and inversely related to ventricular relaxation [59]. Because of intrinsic differences in myocardial fiber orientation, septal Ea velocities are slightly lower than lateral Ea velocities.

In adults over 30 years old, a lateral Ea velocity >12 cm/s is associated with normal LV diastolic function [62] (Fig. 4.4a). Reductions in lateral Ea velocity to ≤8 cm/s in middle-aged to older adults indicate impaired LV relaxation. In cases of restrictive cardiomyopathy, the characteristic intrinsic myocardial abnormalities result in impaired relaxation and reduced Ea velocities.

Peak systolic and early diastolic myocardial tissue velocities have been used to identify early subclinical disease despite normal conventional echocardiographic values in several progressive, nonischemic fibrotic processes [43]. A reduction in both parameters has been detected in patients with diabetes but no evidence of heart failure,

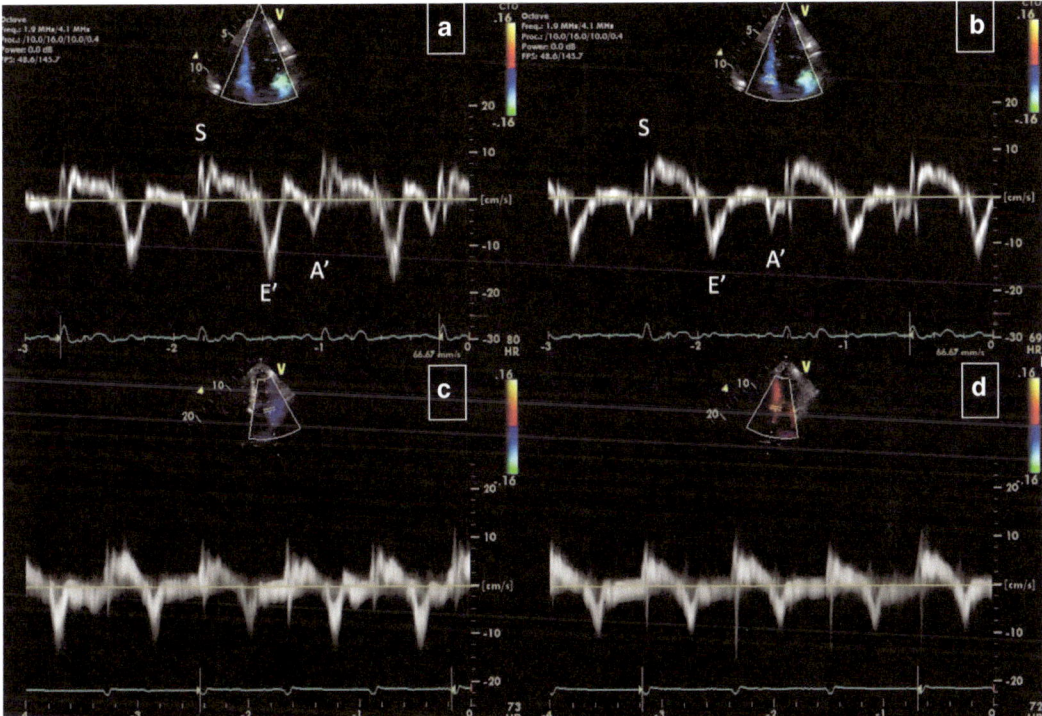

Fig. 4.4 TDI of the lateral (**a**) and septal (**b**) mitral annulus in a normal subject. There are three major velocities: systolic velocity, S′ or Sa, which reflects the systolic function of the left ventricle; E′ or Ea which reflects the status of myocardial relaxation (Normal E′ medial is 10 cm/s and lateral is >15 cm/s); and A′ or Aa is also related to diastolic function of the left ventricle. Panels (**c** and **d**) are from a patient with cardiac amyloidosis and show fusion of the E′ and A′ waves due to underlying atrial fibrillation

and early diastolic tissue velocity has also been found to be reduced with advancing age and hypertension [63]. This impairment in myocardial velocity and resultant impaired ventricular relaxation may reflect interstitial fibrosis, altered cardiomyocyte cytoskeleton properties, or a combination of both. This relationship is supported by endomyocardial biopsy findings that inversely relate percent fibrosis to tissue Doppler-derived systolic and early diastolic tissue velocity [64].

In a recent study of echo versus cardiac MRI post aortic valve replacement (AVR) in patients with severe AS, LGE+ patients had lower E′, S′, and had higher E/E′ [65]. These findings indicate that echo may be used clinically in patients with contraindication to CMR. TDI E′, especially, is a clinically useful clue of risk stratification before AVR in patients with severe AS and preserved LV systolic function. Another study comparing TDI with CMR-LGE imaging showed that subjects with normal diastolic function by TDI exhibited no or minimal fibrosis (median LGE score 0, IQR 0–0) [66]. In contrast, the majority of patients with cardiomyopathy (regardless of etiology) had abnormal diastolic function indices by Doppler echo, and substantial fibrosis (median LGE score 3, IQR 0–6.25). In this study, the prevalence of LGE-positivity by diastolic filling pattern was 13% in normal patients, 48% in impaired relaxation, 78% in pseudo-normal and 87% in restrictive filling pattern (p < 0.0001) [54].

Strain and Strain Rate Imaging

Myocardial velocities measured with TDI can be overestimated by translational motion of the myocardium or underestimated by myocardial tethering. As a result, it is useful to measure the actual extent of myocardial deformation by strain and strain rate imaging. Strain is defined as the change in length of a segment of myocardium relative to its resting length and is expressed as a percentage; strain rate is the rate of this deformation [67]. By convention, shortening is represented by negative values and lengthening by positive values for both strain and strain rate [68]. In a normal individual, longitudinal strain rate values are similar from base to apex. It is possible using a curved cursor during image acquisition, to measure regional strain rate. Ultimately the ultrasound beam needs to be aligned parallel with the direction of myocardial motion. By measuring regional myocardial function, TDI and strain imaging have potential incremental value for the evaluation of cardiomyopathy and diastolic heart failure. Thick myocardial walls due to infiltration or primary cardiomyopathy have reduced TDI and strain values. This is in contrast to normal values obtained in an athlete's heart. It is also useful how the pattern of regional dysfunction can help to identify various underlying cardiomyopathies [69, 70]. In general, global strain measures typically perform better than LVEF in predicting risk [71], and at least two studies suggest that they also offer incremental value beyond clinical information and LVEF [72, 73].

Speckle Tracking Echo

This method quantifies myocardial motion in various planes using 2D images. Reflection, scattering and interference of the ultrasound beam in the myocardial tissue produce a speckle formation [68]. Myocardial regions have unique speckle patterns, which can be tracked from frame to frame throughout the cardiac cycle [69]. Thus an assessment can be made of LV rotational motion, typically referred to as torsion or twist. LV myocardial fibers have a spiral shape, which results in a complex three-dimensional torsion mechanism for systolic contraction and untwisting for diastolic relaxation [74]. The LV subendocardial layer wraps around the LV cavity in the direction of a right-handed helix. In contrast, the subepicardial layer wraps around in the direction of a left-handed helix. When viewed from the LV apex, apical rotation is counterclockwise, and basal rotation is clockwise during systole [68]. Speckle tracking can be used for quantification of LV systolic and potentially diastolic function. In addition, it can be used for measuring strain instead of TDI as discussed above.

Recent work aiming to explore whether LV twist analysis can detect the extent of myocardial fibrosis in patients with hypertrophic cardiomyopathy (HCM) showed that HCM patients had significantly higher basal (Bas)-Rotation, anteroposterior (AP)-Rotation, LV Twist, left ventricular ejection fraction (LVEF), left atrium end systolic dimension (LADs), interventricular septal thickness (IVST), left atrial volume index (LAVi), E/Em and left ventricular mass index (LVMI) than controls (all $p < 0.0001$) and significantly lower left ventricular end-diastolic dimension (LVDd) and E/A (both $p < 0.001$) [75]. The authors concluded that LV twist analysis has good sensitivity and specificity in indicating the severity of myocardial fibrosis in HCM patients [75].

Another study utilizing standard echocardiography, 3-dimensional speckle tracking echocardiography measured peak systolic longitudinal, circumferential, and area strain, LSt, CSt, and ASt, respectively, to quantify LV systolic myocardial mechanics. LGE CMR in HCM patients revealed the area strain as a net result from longitudinal and circumferential deformations. This measurement correlated with functional parameters and the number of significantly hypertrophied segments detected on 2D echo and CMR. All three deformation parameters were attenuated in those myocardial segments with hypertrophy and LGE scar. There was no difference in strain parameters between hypertrophied and LGE segments. They thus concluded that these data demonstrate that hypertrophy seem to be the major independent factors altering global systolic myocardial mechanics in HCM.

In other conditions such as Fabrys disease (FD), it has been proven that fibrosis, as evidenced by the presence of LGE, is associated with lower longitudinal strain (as measured by speckle tracking) in the corresponding fibrotic wall segments [76]. Speckle tracking can thus be used as a tool for the indirect evaluation of LGE and thus myocardial fibrosis in FD. Its use has also been studied in conditions such as severe aortic stenosis [77], and in patients with cardiotoxicity from prior Anthracycline use [78]. In cardiac amyloidosis (CA), speckle tracking echo reveals regional variations in longitudinal strain (LS) from base to apex [79] and with a relative 'apical sparing' pattern of LS, this allows us to differentiate CA from other causes of LV hypertrophy (Figs. 4.5 and 4.6).

In clinical practice, the widespread use of speckle tracking has not been seen to date, likely related to the increased time required for data analysis, however as a research tool it has a fundamental role to play in the evaluation of myocardial fibrosis.

Cardiac Computed Tomography (Multidetector CT)

Cardiac CT thus far has demonstrated initial utility predominantly for the evaluation of myocardial scar. Lardo et al. [80] demonstrated in an animal model that the spatial extent of acute and healed MI could be determined and quantified accurately with contrast-enhanced CT. In this study, the CT findings were compared to histology. Bettencourt et al. [81] found that CT delayed enhancement had good accuracy (90%) for ischemic scar detection with low sensitivity (53%) but

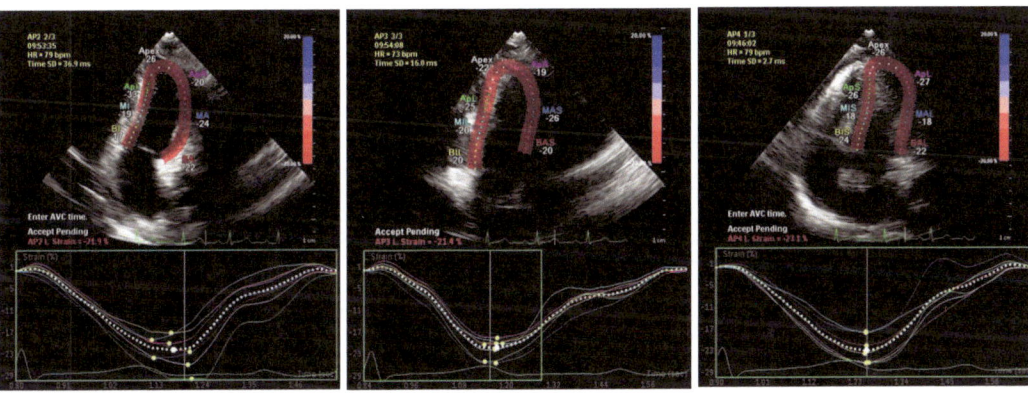

Fig. 4.5 Longitudinal Strain Measurement in a Normal Individual, measured from the 2 chamber view, 3 chamber view and 4 chamber view, respectively, in the same patient (left to right). Shortening is indicated by negative values, which range from −17 to −33, indicating regional variation in a normal heart

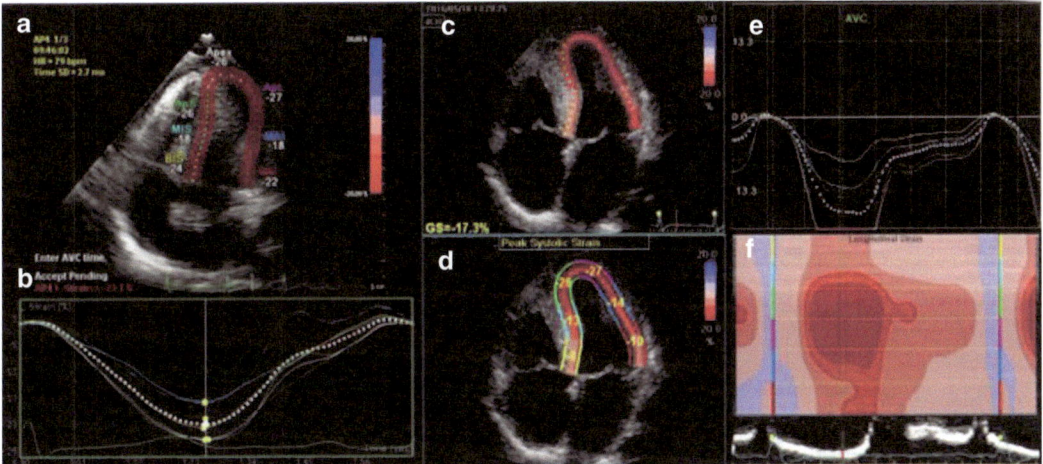

Fig. 4.6 Normal regional and global strain in a normal individual (**a, b**). In contrast the images from panels (**c–f**) are taken from a patient with cardiac amyloidosis. There is abnormal longitudinal strain affecting the basal segments with relative sparing of the apical segments and reduced overall global longitudinal strain

excellent specificity (98%). The use of MDCT for diffuse abnormalities of myocardial tissue is significantly more challenging than the evaluation of focal myocardial scar due to the low contrast resolution of CT scanning [82]. ECV measured with cardiac CT represents a novel approach toward the clinical assessment of diffuse myocardial fibrosis. It has been shown that there is a good correlation between myocardial ECV measured with cardiac CT and with T1 map measured by cardiac MR imaging in 24 subjects [83]. This study included patients with heart failure and normal controls and showed that ECV was higher in patients with heart failure for both cardiac CT and cardiac MR imaging. Also, for both cardiac MR and cardiac CT, ECV was positively associated with end diastolic and end systolic volumes and inversely related to ejection fraction (EF).

Additional supportive data for MDCT comes from Bandula et al. [84] who demonstrated that ECV measured using a equilibrium CT technique in patients with aortic stenosis correlated well with histologic quantification of myocardial fibrosis, and also with ECV derived by using equilibrium MR imaging. From a clinical perspective, MDCT has also been studied in hypertrophic cardiomyopathy [85] and found to reliably detect myocardial fibrosis as evident by LGE. Patient- and segment-based sensitivity was 100% and 68%, respectively, compared to LGE-CMR. In patients with a contraindication to CMR, this technique could therefore be useful.

Conclusion

The use of noninvasive imaging methods of myocardial fibrosis has increased in recent years. Exciting and novel techniques will continue to emerge in the years to come. Cardiac MRI has proven to be an important tool through the use of LGE-CMR and T1 mapping techniques, both in the clinical and research arena. Clinically it is now possible to carry out a full study and answer the question regarding the presence or absence of underlying myocardial fibrosis in under 45 min. In the presence of claustrophobia, non-CMR compatible devices, and inability to breath hold, alternative imaging techniques must be considered. Echo is a reliable clinical and research tool, which has been well validated in this area. Nuclear techniques for detection of myocardial scar and myocardial viability play an important role in clinical practice. Molecular techniques are still very much research tools but are promising for future use in this field. MDCT has also proven its use as described above although the radiation dose makes it a less attractive option.

Overall, cardiac MRI has a proven benefit in the detection of underlying myocardial fibrosis. It is hoped that with earlier detection, therapies may be developed to tackle myocardial disease prior to the development of heart failure symptoms and signs.

References

1. de Haas HJ, Arbustini E, Fuster V, Kramer CM, Narula J. Molecular imaging of the cardiac extracellular matrix. Circ Res. 2014;114(5):903–15.
2. Weber KT, Janicki JS, Shroff SG, Pick R, Chen RM, Bashey RI. Collagen remodeling of the pressure-overloaded, hypertrophied nonhuman primate myocardium. Circ Res. 1988;62(4):757–65.
3. Borer JS, Truter S, Herrold EM, Falcone DJ, Pena M, Carter JN, et al. Myocardial fibrosis in chronic aortic regurgitation: molecular and cellular responses to volume overload. Circulation. 2002;105(15):1837–42.
4. Tanaka M, Fujiwara H, Onodera T, Wu DJ, Hamashima Y, Kawai C. Quantitative analysis of myocardial fibrosis in normals, hypertensive hearts, and hypertrophic cardiomyopathy. Br Heart J. 1986;55(6):575–81.
5. Tandri H, Saranathan M, Rodriguez ER, Martinez C, Bomma C, Nasir K, et al. Noninvasive detection of myocardial fibrosis in arrhythmogenic right ventricular cardiomyopathy using delayed-enhancement magnetic resonance imaging. J Am Coll Cardiol. 2005;45(1):98–103.
6. Assomull RG, Prasad SK, Lyne J, Smith G, Burman ED, Khan M, et al. Cardiovascular magnetic resonance, fibrosis, and prognosis in dilated cardiomyopathy. J Am Coll Cardiol. 2006;48(10):1977–85.
7. van den Borne SW, Isobe S, Verjans JW, Petrov A, Lovhaug D, Li P, et al. Molecular imaging of interstitial alterations in remodeling myocardium after myocardial infarction. J Am Coll Cardiol. 2008;52(24):2017–28.
8. Martos R, Baugh J, Ledwidge M, O'Loughlin C, Conlon C, Patle A, et al. Diastolic heart failure: evidence of increased myocardial collagen turnover linked to diastolic dysfunction. Circulation. 2007;115(7):888–95.

9. Mewton N, Liu CY, Croisille P, Bluemke D, Lima JA. Assessment of myocardial fibrosis with cardiovascular magnetic resonance. J Am Coll Cardiol. 2011;57(8):891–903.

10. Mahrholdt H, Goedecke C, Wagner A, Meinhardt G, Athanasiadis A, Vogelsberg H, et al. Cardiovascular magnetic resonance assessment of human myocarditis: a comparison to histology and molecular pathology. Circulation. 2004;109(10):1250–8.

11. Bocchi EA, Kalil R, Bacal F, de Lourdes Higuchi M, Meneghetti C, Magalhaes A, et al. Magnetic resonance imaging in chronic chagas' disease: correlation with endomyocardial biopsy findings and gallium-67 cardiac uptake. Echocardiography. 1998;15(3):279–88.

12. Kim RJ, Chen EL, Lima JA, Judd RM. Myocardial Gd-DTPA kinetics determine MRI contrast enhancement and reflect the extent and severity of myocardial injury after acute reperfused infarction. Circulation. 1996;94(12):3318–26.

13. Debl K, Djavidani B, Buchner S, Lipke C, Nitz W, Feuerbach S, et al. Delayed hyperenhancement in magnetic resonance imaging of left ventricular hypertrophy caused by aortic stenosis and hypertrophic cardiomyopathy: visualisation of focal fibrosis. Heart. 2006;92(10):1447–51.

14. De Cobelli F, Pieroni M, Esposito A, Chimenti C, Belloni E, Mellone R, et al. Delayed gadolinium-enhanced cardiac magnetic resonance in patients with chronic myocarditis presenting with heart failure or recurrent arrhythmias. J Am Coll Cardiol. 2006;47(8):1649–54.

15. Choudhury L, Mahrholdt H, Wagner A, Choi KM, Elliott MD, Klocke FJ, et al. Myocardial scarring in asymptomatic or mildly symptomatic patients with hypertrophic cardiomyopathy. J Am Coll Cardiol. 2002;40(12):2156–64.

16. McCrohon JA, Moon JC, Prasad SK, McKenna WJ, Lorenz CH, Coats AJ, et al. Differentiation of heart failure related to dilated cardiomyopathy and coronary artery disease using gadolinium-enhanced cardiovascular magnetic resonance. Circulation. 2003;108(1):54–9.

17. Mahrholdt H, Wagner A, Judd RM, Sechtem U, Kim RJ. Delayed enhancement cardiovascular magnetic resonance assessment of non-ischaemic cardiomyopathies. Eur Heart J. 2005;26(15):1461–74.

18. Rehwald WG, Fieno DS, Chen EL, Kim RJ, Judd RM. Myocardial magnetic resonance imaging contrast agent concentrations after reversible and irreversible ischemic injury. Circulation. 2002;105(2):224–9.

19. Croisille P, Revel D, Saeed M. Contrast agents and cardiac MR imaging of myocardial ischemia: from bench to bedside. Eur Radiol. 2006;16(9):1951–63.

20. Messroghli DR, Radjenovic A, Kozerke S, Higgins DM, Sivananthan MU, Ridgway JP. Modified look-locker inversion recovery (MOLLI) for high-resolution T1 mapping of the heart. Magn Reson Med. 2004;52(1):141–6.

21. Piechnik SK, Ferreira VM, Dall'Armellina E, Cochlin LE, Greiser A, Neubauer S, et al. Shortened modified look-locker Inversion recovery (ShMOLLI) for clinical myocardial T1-mapping at 1.5 and 3 T within a 9 heartbeat breathhold. J Cardiovasc Magn Reson. 2010;12:69.

22. Robbers LF, Baars EN, Brouwer WP, Beek AM, Hofman MB, Niessen HW, et al. T1 mapping shows increased extracellular matrix size in the myocardium due to amyloid depositions. Circ Cardiovasc Imaging. 2012;5(3):423–6.

23. Iles L, Pfluger H, Phrommintikul A, Cherayath J, Aksit P, Gupta SN, et al. Evaluation of diffuse myocardial fibrosis in heart failure with cardiac magnetic resonance contrast-enhanced T1 mapping. J Am Coll Cardiol. 2008;52(19):1574–80.

24. Sibley CT, Noureldin RA, Gai N, Nacif MS, Liu S, Turkbey EB, et al. T1 mapping in cardiomyopathy at cardiac MR: comparison with endomyocardial biopsy. Radiology. 2012;265(3):724–32.

25. Messroghli DR, Niendorf T, Schulz-Menger J, Dietz R, Friedrich MG. T1 mapping in patients with acute myocardial infarction. J Cardiovasc Magn Reson. 2003;5(2):353–9.

26. Maceira AM, Joshi J, Prasad SK, Moon JC, Perugini E, Harding I, et al. Cardiovascular magnetic resonance in cardiac amyloidosis. Circulation. 2005;111(2):186–93.

27. Messroghli DR, Walters K, Plein S, Sparrow P, Friedrich MG, Ridgway JP, et al. Myocardial T1 mapping: application to patients with acute and chronic myocardial infarction. Magn Reson Med. 2007;58(1):34–40.

28. Broberg CS, Chugh SS, Conklin C, Sahn DJ, Jerosch-Herold M. Quantification of diffuse myocardial fibrosis and its association with myocardial dysfunction in congenital heart disease. Circ Cardiovasc Imaging. 2010;3(6):727–34.

29. Flett AS, Hayward MP, Ashworth MT, Hansen MS, Taylor AM, Elliott PM, et al. Equilibrium contrast cardiovascular magnetic resonance for the measurement of diffuse myocardial fibrosis: preliminary validation in humans. Circulation. 2010;122(2):138–44.

30. Gai N, Turkbey EB, Nazarian S, van der Geest RJ, Liu CY, Lima JA, et al. T1 mapping of the gadolinium-enhanced myocardium: adjustment for factors affecting interpatient comparison. Magn Reson Med. 2011;65(5):1407–15.

31. Bauner KU, Biffar A, Theisen D, Greiser A, Zech CJ, Nguyen ET, et al. Extracellular volume fractions in chronic myocardial infarction. Investig Radiol. 2012;47(9):538–45.

32. Turkbey EB, Gai N, Lima JA, van der Geest RJ, Wagner KR, Tomaselli GF, et al. Assessment of cardiac involvement in myotonic muscular dystrophy by T1 mapping on magnetic resonance imaging. Heart Rhythm. 2012;9(10):1691–7.

33. Dass S, Suttie JJ, Piechnik SK, Ferreira VM, Holloway CJ, Banerjee R, et al. Myocardial tissue characterization using magnetic resonance noncontrast t1 mapping in hypertrophic and dilated cardiomyopathy. Circ Cardiovasc Imaging. 2012;5(6):726–33.

34. Fontana M, White SK, Banypersad SM, Sado DM, Maestrini V, Flett AS, et al. Comparison of T1 mapping techniques for ECV quantification. Histological validation and reproducibility of ShMOLLI versus multibreath-hold T1 quantification equilibrium contrast CMR. J Cardiovasc Magn Reson. 2012;14:88.

35. Rao AD, Shah RV, Garg R, Abbasi SA, Neilan TG, Perlstein TS, et al. Aldosterone and myocardial extracellular matrix expansion in type 2 diabetes mellitus. Am J Cardiol. 2013;112(1):73–8.

36. Ellims AH, Shaw JA, Stub D, Iles LM, Hare JL, Slavin GS, et al. Diffuse myocardial fibrosis evaluated by post-contrast t1 mapping correlates with left ventricular stiffness. J Am Coll Cardiol. 2014;63(11):1112–8.

37. Schulz-Menger J, Bluemke DA, Bremerich J, Flamm SD, Fogel MA, Friedrich MG, et al. Standardized image interpretation and post processing in cardiovascular magnetic resonance: Society for Cardiovascular Magnetic Resonance (SCMR) board of trustees task force on standardized post processing. J Cardiovasc Magn Reson. 2013;15:35.

38. Gatehouse PD, Bydder GM. Magnetic resonance imaging of short T2 components in tissue. Clin Radiol. 2003;58(1):1–19.

39. de Jong S, Zwanenburg JJ, Visser F, der Nagel R, van Rijen HV, Vos MA, et al. Direct detection of myocardial fibrosis by MRI. J Mol Cell Cardiol. 2011;51(6):974–9.

40. Siu AG, Ramadeen A, Hu X, Morikawa L, Zhang L, Lau JY, et al. Characterization of the ultrashort-TE (UTE) MR collagen signal. NMR Biomed. 2015;28(10):1236–44.

41. Vandsburger M, Vandoorne K, Oren R, Leftin A, Mpofu S, Delli Castelli D, et al. Cardio-chemical exchange saturation transfer magnetic resonance imaging reveals molecular signatures of endogenous fibrosis and exogenous contrast media. Circ Cardiovasc Imaging. 2015;8(1).

42. Helm PA, Caravan P, French BA, Jacques V, Shen L, Xu Y, et al. Postinfarction myocardial scarring in mice: molecular MR imaging with use of a collagen-targeting contrast agent. Radiology. 2008;247(3):788–96.

43. Jellis C, Martin J, Narula J, Marwick TH. Assessment of nonischemic myocardial fibrosis. J Am Coll Cardiol. 2010;56(2):89–97.

44. Yamamoto Y, de Silva R, Rhodes CG, Araujo LI, Iida H, Rechavia E, et al. A new strategy for the assessment of viable myocardium and regional myocardial blood flow using 15O-water and dynamic positron emission tomography. Circulation. 1992;86(1):167–78.

45. Knaapen P, Boellaard R, Gotte MJ, Dijkmans PA, van Campen LM, de Cock CC, et al. Perfusable tissue index as a potential marker of fibrosis in patients with idiopathic dilated cardiomyopathy. J Nucl Med. 2004;45(8):1299–304.

46. Knaapen P, Gotte MJ, Paulus WJ, Zwanenburg JJ, Dijkmans PA, Boellaard R, et al. Does myocardial fibrosis hinder contractile function and perfusion in idiopathic dilated cardiomyopathy? PET and MR imaging study. Radiology. 2006;240(2):380–8.

47. Knaapen P, van Dockum WG, Bondarenko O, Kok WE, Gotte MJ, Boellaard R, et al. Delayed contrast enhancement and perfusable tissue index in hypertrophic cardiomyopathy: comparison between cardiac MRI and PET. J Nucl Med. 2005;46(6):923–9.

48. van den Borne SW, Isobe S, Zandbergen HR, Li P, Petrov A, Wong ND, et al. Molecular imaging for efficacy of pharmacologic intervention in myocardial remodeling. JACC Cardiovasc Imaging. 2009;2(2):187–98.

49. Tadamura E, Kudoh T, Hattori N, Inubushi M, Magata Y, Konishi J, et al. Impairment of BMIPP uptake precedes abnormalities in oxygen and glucose metabolism in hypertrophic cardiomyopathy. J Nucl Med. 1998;39(3):390–6.

50. Delgado V, Bax JJ. Clinical topic: Nuclear imaging in hypertrophic cardiomyopathy. J Nucl Cardiol. 2015;22(3):408–18.

51. Hashimura H, Kiso K, Yamada N, Kono A, Morita Y, Fukushima K, et al. Myocardial impairment detected by late gadolinium enhancement in hypertrophic cardiomyopathy: comparison with 99mTc-MIBI/tetrofosmin and 123I-BMIPP SPECT. Kobe J Med Sci. 2013;59(3):E81–92.

52. Mimbs JW, O'Donnell M, Bauwens D, Miller JW, Sobel BE. The dependence of ultrasonic attenuation and backscatter on collagen content in dog and rabbit hearts. Circ Res. 1980;47(1):49–58.

53. Shapiro LM, Moore RB, Logan-Sinclair RB, Gibson DG. Relation of regional echo amplitude to left ventricular function and the electrocardiogram in left ventricular hypertrophy. Br Heart J. 1984;52(1):99–105.

54. Picano E, Pelosi G, Marzilli M, Lattanzi F, Benassi A, Landini L, et al. In vivo quantitative ultrasonic evaluation of myocardial fibrosis in humans. Circulation. 1990;81(1):58–64.

55. Lin YH, Shiau YC, Yen RF, Lin LC, Wu CC, Ho YL, et al. The relation between myocardial cyclic variation of integrated backscatter and serum concentrations of procollagen propeptides in hypertensive patients. Ultrasound Med Biol. 2004;30(7):885–91.

56. Naito J, Masuyama T, Mano T, Kondo H, Yamamoto K, Nagano R, et al. Analysis of transmural trend of myocardial integrated ultrasonic backscatter in patients with old myocardial infarction. Ultrasound Med Biol. 1996;22(7):807–14.

57. Fang ZY, Leano R, Marwick TH. Relationship between longitudinal and radial contractility in subclinical diabetic heart disease. Clin Sci (Lond). 2004;106(1):53–60.

58. Mele D, Censi S, La Corte R, Merli E, Lo Monaco A, Locaputo A, et al. Abnormalities of left ventricular function in asymptomatic patients with systemic sclerosis using Doppler measures of myocardial strain. J Am Soc Echocardiogr. 2008;21(11):1257–64.

59. Ho CY, Solomon SD. A clinician's guide to tissue Doppler imaging. Circulation. 2006;113(10):e396–8.

60. Vinereanu D, Khokhar A, Fraser AG. Reproducibility of pulsed wave tissue Doppler echocardiography. J Am Soc Echocardiogr. 1999;12(6):492–9.

61. Galiuto L, Ignone G, DeMaria AN. Contraction and relaxation velocities of the normal left ventricle using

pulsed-wave tissue Doppler echocardiography. Am J Cardiol. 1998;81(5):609–14.

62. Yamada H, Oki T, Mishiro Y, Tabata T, Abe M, Onose Y, et al. Effect of aging on diastolic left ventricular myocardial velocities measured by pulsed tissue Doppler imaging in healthy subjects. J Am Soc Echocardiogr. 1999;12(7):574–81.

63. Fang ZY, Schull-Meade R, Downey M, Prins J, Marwick TH. Determinants of subclinical diabetic heart disease. Diabetologia. 2005;48(2):394–402.

64. Shan K, Bick RJ, Poindexter BJ, Shimoni S, Letsou GV, Reardon MJ, et al. Relation of tissue Doppler derived myocardial velocities to myocardial structure and beta-adrenergic receptor density in humans. J Am Coll Cardiol. 2000;36(3):891–6.

65. Park J, Chang HJ, Choi JH, Yang PS, Lee SE, Heo R, et al. Late gadolinium enhancement in cardiac MRI in patients with severe aortic stenosis and preserved left ventricular systolic function is related to attenuated improvement of left ventricular geometry and filling pressure after aortic valve replacement. Korean Circ J. 2014;44(5):312–9.

66. Moreo A, Ambrosio G, De Chiara B, Pu M, Tran T, Mauri F, et al. Influence of myocardial fibrosis on left ventricular diastolic function: noninvasive assessment by cardiac magnetic resonance and echo. Circ Cardiovasc Imaging. 2009;2(6):437–43.

67. Shah AM, Solomon SD. Myocardial deformation imaging: current status and future directions. Circulation. 2012;125(2):e244–8.

68. Oh JK, James Seward JB, Tajik AJ. The echo manual. 3rd ed. Philadelphia: Lippincott Williams & Wilkins; 2007.

69. Helle-Valle T, Crosby J, Edvardsen T, Lyseggen E, Amundsen BH, Smith HJ, et al. New noninvasive method for assessment of left ventricular rotation: speckle tracking echocardiography. Circulation. 2005;112(20):3149–56.

70. Masci PG, Marinelli M, Piacenti M, Lorenzoni V, Positano V, Lombardi M, et al. Myocardial structural, perfusion, and metabolic correlates of left bundle branch block mechanical derangement in patients with dilated cardiomyopathy: a tagged cardiac magnetic resonance and positron emission tomography study. Circ Cardiovasc Imaging. 2010;3(4):482–90.

71. Nahum J, Bensaid A, Dussault C, Macron L, Clemence D, Bouhemad B, et al. Impact of longitudinal myocardial deformation on the prognosis of chronic heart failure patients. Circ Cardiovasc Imaging. 2010;3(3):249–56.

72. Hung CL, Verma A, Uno H, Shin SH, Bourgoun M, Hassanein AH, et al. Longitudinal and circumferential strain rate, left ventricular remodeling, and prognosis after myocardial infarction. J Am Coll Cardiol. 2010;56(22):1812–22.

73. Cho GY, Marwick TH, Kim HS, Kim MK, Hong KS, Oh DJ. Global 2-dimensional strain as a new prognosticator in patients with heart failure. J Am Coll Cardiol. 2009;54(7):618–24.

74. Sengupta PP, Khandheria BK, Korinek J, Wang J, Jahangir A, Seward JB, et al. Apex-to-base dispersion in regional timing of left ventricular shortening and lengthening. J Am Coll Cardiol. 2006;47(1):163–72.

75. Zhang HJ, Wang H, Sun T, Lu MJ, Xu N, Wu WC, et al. Assessment of left ventricular twist mechanics by speckle tracking echocardiography reveals association between LV twist and myocardial fibrosis in patients with hypertrophic cardiomyopathy. Int J Cardiovasc Imaging. 2014;30(8):1539–48.

76. Kramer J, Niemann M, Liu D, Hu K, Machann W, Beer M, et al. Two-dimensional speckle tracking as a non-invasive tool for identification of myocardial fibrosis in Fabry disease. Eur Heart J. 2013;34(21):1587–96.

77. Hoffmann R, Altiok E, Friedman Z, Becker M, Frick M. Myocardial deformation imaging by two-dimensional speckle-tracking echocardiography in comparison to late gadolinium enhancement cardiac magnetic resonance for analysis of myocardial fibrosis in severe aortic stenosis. Am J Cardiol. 2014;114(7):1083–8.

78. Ho E, Brown A, Barrett P, Morgan RB, King G, Kennedy MJ, et al. Subclinical anthracycline- and trastuzumab-induced cardiotoxicity in the long-term follow-up of asymptomatic breast cancer survivors: a speckle tracking echocardiographic study. Heart. 2010;96(9):701–7.

79. Phelan D, Collier P, Thavendiranathan P, Popovic ZB, Hanna M, Plana JC, et al. Relative apical sparing of longitudinal strain using two-dimensional speckle-tracking echocardiography is both sensitive and specific for the diagnosis of cardiac amyloidosis. Heart. 2012;98(19):1442–8.

80. Lardo AC, Cordeiro MA, Silva C, Amado LC, George RT, Saliaris AP, et al. Contrast-enhanced multidetector computed tomography viability imaging after myocardial infarction: characterization of myocyte death, microvascular obstruction, and chronic scar. Circulation. 2006;113(3):394–404.

81. Bettencourt N, Rocha J, Carvalho M, Leite D, Toschke AM, Melica B, et al. Multislice computed tomography in the exclusion of coronary artery disease in patients with presurgical valve disease. Circ Cardiovasc Imaging. 2009;2(4):306–13.

82. Pattanayak P, Bleumke DA. Tissue characterization of the myocardium: state of the art characterization by magnetic resonance and computed tomography imaging. Radiol Clin N Am. 2015;53(2):413–23.

83. Nacif MS, Kawel N, Lee JJ, Chen X, Yao J, Zavodni A, et al. Interstitial myocardial fibrosis assessed as extracellular volume fraction with low-radiation-dose cardiac CT. Radiology. 2012;264(3):876–83.

84. Bandula S, White SK, Flett AS, Lawrence D, Pugliese F, Ashworth MT, et al. Measurement of myocardial extracellular volume fraction by using equilibrium contrast-enhanced CT: validation against histologic findings. Radiology. 2013;269(2):396–403.

85. Langer C, Lutz M, Eden M, Ludde M, Hohnhorst M, Gierloff C, et al. Hypertrophic cardiomyopathy in cardiac CT: a validation study on the detection of intramyocardial fibrosis in consecutive patients. Int J Cardiovasc Imaging. 2014;30(3):659–67.

T1 Mapping in Aortic Stenosis

Russell J. Everett, David E. Newby, and Marc R. Dweck

Epidemiology

Aortic stenosis is the most clinically important valve disease in the Western world and is set to triple by 2050 [1, 2]. Calcification and stenosis of the valve lead to progressive left ventricular hypertrophy (LVH) and ultimately left ventricular (LV) decompensation and heart failure (HF) unless aortic valve (AV) replacement surgery is performed (Fig. 5.1).

Natural History

Current clinical guidelines advise AV replacement in the presence of symptoms (exertional angina, syncope or dyspnoea) or impairment of left ventricular ejection fraction. This recommendation is, however, based on studies dating back to the 1960s, showing poor prognosis following symptom development in a middle-aged patient population with bicuspid or rheumatic heart disease [3]. The demographics of aortic stenosis have since shifted with most patients developing calcific disease of tri-leaflet valves. In addition, patients are now usually elderly with multiple comorbidities, which may confound the valvular

etiology of the symptoms. The development of a reduced left ventricular ejection fraction (LVEF <50% on echocardiographic assessment), while undoubtedly portending a poor prognosis [4, 5], is now recognised as an insensitive marker of LV decompensation and is often irreversible following AV replacement [4]. The identification of other more sensitive markers of LV decompensation or adverse prognosis is, therefore, desirable.

Clinical Presentation

Aortic stenosis (AS) is diagnosed in the majority of patients after the incidental detection of a systolic ejection murmur on clinical examination. The diagnosis is then confirmed on transthoracic echocardiography. The classical symptoms of AS are exertional chest pain, dyspnea and syncope but they do not manifest themselves until the disease is very advanced and severe valve narrowing has developed. Even then, the correlation between the valve gradient and symptoms is weak, suggesting other factors, such as the LV myocardial response to pressure overload, which are important in determining symptomatology and the natural history of the condition.

R. J. Everett (✉) · D. E. Newby · M. R. Dweck
British Heart Foundation Centre for Cardiovascular Science, University of Edinburgh, Edinburgh, UK
e-mail: D.E.Newby@ed.ac.uk;
mdweck@staffmail.ed.ac.uk

P. C. Yang (ed.), *T1-Mapping in Myocardial Disease*, https://doi.org/10.1007/978-3-319-91110-6_5

Fig. 5.1 Progression from left ventricular hypertrophy in aortic stenosis. Progressive aortic valve narrowing results in increased left ventricular (LV) wall stress due to increased afterload. This results in increasing LV hypertrophy which normalizes wall stress. However, this process ultimately decompensates with mid-wall myocardial fibrosis (black arrow) secondary to direct wall stress, myocardial ischemia and the effects of angiotensin. If pressure overload is not alleviated with aortic valve intervention, heart failure and death ensue. *LV* left ventricular

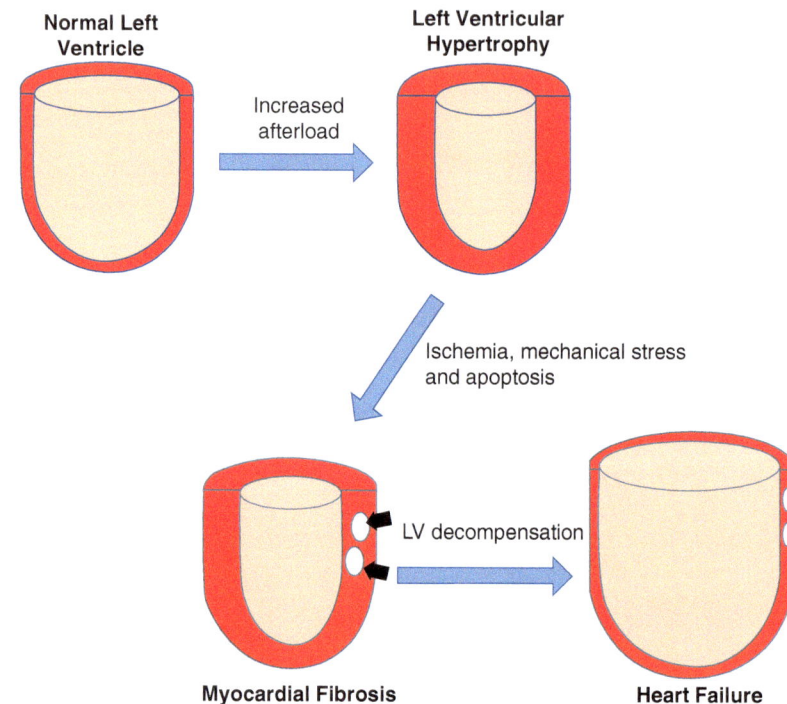

Pathobiology of Valvular Disease

Our understanding of the pathophysiology of AS has progressed significantly in recent years, and a disease that was once thought to be caused by degenerative "wear and tear" of the valve has been shown to comprise a highly regulated process of inflammation, calcification and fibrosis (Fig. 5.2) [6]. The early stages of aortic stenosis are thought to be similar to atherosclerosis with predominantly endothelial damage and inflammatory response. This is due to the increased wall stress and reduced sheer stress, which is highest around the flexion areas of the cusps adjacent to aortic root attachment where most AS lesions are observed. Both cusp tips and commissures are also frequently involved with lesions usually occurring in the fibrosa layer on the aortic aspect of the valve. Endothelial damage and lipid deposition trigger inflammation within the AV, resulting in an inflammatory cell infiltrate. One of the best ways of noninvasively assessing the presence of inflammation is with 18F-fluorodeoxyglucose positron emission tomography (PET) and computed tomography (CT). There have been few studies so far in this area but 18F-fluorodeoxyglucose uptake is detectable *in vivo* and is increased in patients with AS compared to controls with a correlation between PET signal intensity and AS severity [7].

This inflammation is further sustained by angiogenesis in the valve tissue. Thin neovessels can be seen in the areas of inflammation in the calcific valves, which express a variety of intracellular adhesion molecules and suggest their role in point of entry for inflammatory cells. These neovessels are frequently associated with hemorrhage and accelerated disease progression.

Over time, inflammation appears to progress to fibrosis. This occurs as a subset of the valve interstitial cells, the predominant cellular component of valve tissue, which differentiate into myofibroblasts under the influence of inflammatory signaling molecules. These myofibroblasts then secrete matrix metalloproteinases (MMP), which are thought to play a role in restructuring the extracellular matrix (ECM) of the valve, leading to accumulation of ECM components, predominantly collagen types I and III (Fig. 5.3). This leads to valve thickening and increased stiffness.

Fig. 5.2 Picrosirius red staining of myocardial biopsies in patients with aortic stenosis. Histological samples examined with light microscopy (×20) (right-sided images) and auto-generated color threshold masks (left-sided images). The first patient has minimal myocardial fibrosis (**a**) whereas advanced fibrosis is present in the second (**b**)

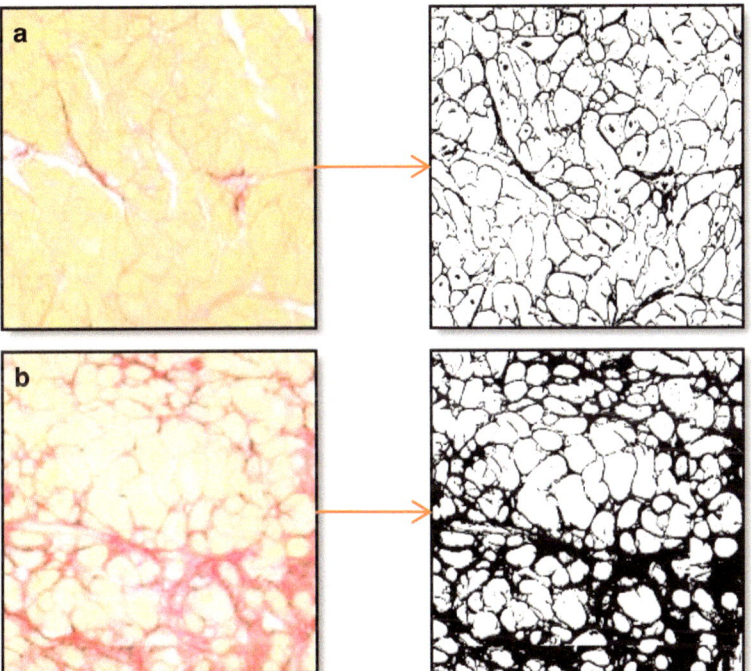

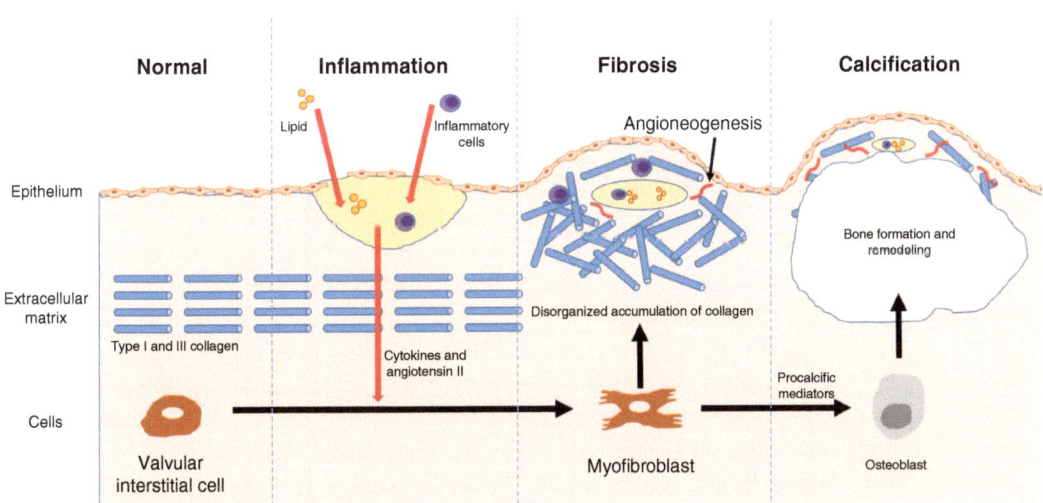

Fig. 5.3 Summary of the pathological processes occurring within the valve during aortic stenosis. Mechanical stress results in endothelial damage that allows infiltration of lipid and inflammatory cells into the valve. Lipid oxidization further increases inflammatory activity within these lesions and the secretion of pro-inflammatory and -fibrotic cytokines. The latter drives the differentiation of fibroblasts into myofibroblasts that secrete increased collagen. Disorganized fibrous tissue accumulates within the valve leading to thickening and increased stiffness of the valve. Myofibroblast differentiation into osteoblasts occurs under the influence of several pro-calcific pathways. Osteoblasts, subsequently, coordinate calcification of the valve as part of a highly regulated process akin to skeletal bone formation with expression of many of the same mediators. These pathogenic processes are sustained by angiogenesis with new vessels localizing, in particular, to regions of inflammation surrounding calcific deposits

The final pathological process in most patients appears to be valvular calcification, which is thought to be driven by the differentiation of myofibroblasts into osteoblasts under the control of a variety of cellular signalling pathways. This leads to progressive calcification similar to skeletal bone formation with the production of a number of osteogenic signaling proteins, resulting in increasing valve stenosis. Once established, the presence of active calcification appears to beget further calcification leading to rapid disease progression in what is termed the "propagation" phase.

There are no effective medical treatments to date that slow or reverse the pathological processes occurring in the valve. Given the similarities with atherosclerosis in the early phases of AS (lipid accumulation and inflammation), it was postulated that cholesterol modifying therapies may have been effective in slowing disease progression. However, three trials of statin therapy all failed to show benefit [8–10].

Patients with osteoporosis have increased severity of aortic stenosis and faster disease progression. Given that both conditions express abnormalities of calcium metabolism, treatments for osteoporosis such as bisphosphonates and denosumab may have a beneficial effect in AS. This is currently being examined in the SALTIRE 2 randomised controlled trial (NCT02132026).

Pathobiology of LV Remodeling

Significant pathological changes occur in the LV as a consequence of progressive increases in afterload and left ventricular wall stress due to valvular stenosis. Left ventricular hypertrophy occurs as an adaptive response to increasing afterload, characterised by myocyte enlargement and LV wall thickening. This initially normalises LV wall stress; however, this process eventually becomes maladaptive, leading to LV decompensation and HF.

Myocyte hypertrophy is accompanied by expansion of the extracellular network of capillaries, nerves and support fibres, comprising the ECM. The increase in capillary density is, however, insufficient to meet the metabolic demands of the hypertrophied myocardium, and coronary flow is further attenuated by increases in coronary vascular resistance due to increased LV transmural pressure. This leads to myocardial ischaemia and a net loss of myocytes due to increase in the rates of cell death by apoptosis. Angiotensin II may also be implicated in this process as studies have shown that angiotensin receptor blockers can inhibit apoptosis in patients with hypertension.

Myocardial Fibrosis

The growth in extracellular matrix itself also becomes maladaptive, similar to that occurring in valve tissue. Myofibroblasts produce extracellular matrix components, predominantly collagen type I and III, which are deposited in the interstitial space [11]. This is thought to be driven by factors similar to those that occur in the valve tissue, namely increases in transforming growth factor beta, angiotensin and relative imbalance in matrix metalloproteinases compared to their inhibitors.

This homogenous increase in extracellular matrix is termed diffuse fibrosis and can be appreciated on histological analysis of myocardial biopsy samples in aortic stenosis patients. This is usually assessed, using picrosirius red or fibronectin staining, and enables automated quantification of fibrosis expressed as a percentage of the myocardial area on the slide, sometimes termed "collagen volume fraction". Progressive accumulation of diffuse fibrosis is associated with increase in LV end-diastolic pressure, impairment in LV diastolic function and ejection fraction [11] and adverse clinical outcomes [12].

Fibrosis appears to co-localise to areas of focal myocyte apoptosis. It has been suggested that this "replacement fibrosis" occurs in areas of scarring, following myocyte cell death, and represents end-stage progression from diffuse fibrosis. Moreover, it is a strong independent predictor of adverse outcome in aortic stenosis and is irreversible, following relief of pressure overload with aortic valve intervention.

In contrast, there is evidence that diffuse fibrosis may regress following AV replacement. In an early longitudinal pathological study, Krayenbeuhl and colleagues investigated 27 patients with severe aortic stenosis, awaiting valve replacement, who underwent invasive angiography with endomyocardial biopsy [13]. Twenty-three patients underwent repeat study with biopsy 18 months following surgery and 9 of these patients were re-biopsied at an average of 70 months following aortic valve replacement. There was significantly more histological fibrosis in patients with aortic stenosis compared to controls (18.2 ± 6.2% versus 7.0 ± 1.8%). As expected, 18 months following aortic valve replacement both the volume and mass measurements decreased consistent with regression of the left ventricular hypertrophic response, following relief of pressure overload. Interestingly they were able to show this was predominantly due to regression of cellular hypertrophy with no change in absolute fibrosis volume in the heart. As a result, diffuse fibrosis measured as a percentage of the myocardial mass actually *increased* in the initial post-operative period. However, on later long-term (6–7 years) re-examination following aortic valve replacement, the percentage diffuse fibrosis had fallen and the absolute fibrosis volume had decreased. It, therefore, appears that diffuse fibrosis is reversible but that regression may take years and be delayed compared to the observed resolution in hypertrophy.

This is the only histological study that provides us with a guide to possible timeframe of diffuse fibrosis regression following AV replacement in AS. Using T1 mapping, Flett and colleagues examined 63 patients with severe aortic stenosis, 42 had repeat imaging 6 months post AV replacement. These results mirrored the above histological study showing regression in myocardial mass at 6 months but with no reduction in myocardial fibrosis [14]. We currently lack studies to examine regression in diffuse fibrosis longitudinally.

Left ventricular hypertrophy and myocardial fibrosis appear crucial to the development of symptoms and adverse events, which are poorly predicted from assessment of AS severity alone. This reinforces that importance of evaluation of the health of the LV myocardium alongside traditional measures of AS severity.

Investigations

Electrocardiography

The 12-lead electrocardiogram (ECG) is useful in the assessment of patients with AS. Although unable to directly detect valve stenosis, the secondary left ventricular hypertrophy leads to characteristic ECG changes, which are specific but poorly sensitive for the presence of significant left ventricular hypertrophy. These include left axis deviation, increasing QRS voltage in both chest and limb leads, change in ST or T wave vector, and broadening of the QRS duration. Furthermore, the presence of ST depression in the lateral leads, representing LV strain, has been shown to predict increased LV mass, high-sensitivity troponin value, and mid-wall replacement fibrosis (positive predictive value 100%) [15]. The ECG-strain pattern is also a powerful predictor of adverse events in AS.

Echocardiography

Echocardiography is the cornerstone of assessment for aortic stenosis and has almost entirely supplanted invasive catheter-based assessment. It is non-invasive, safe, relatively inexpensive and widely available. In particular, echocardiography enables detailed assessment of AV morphology and function both by visual and Doppler assessment. Severity of valvular stenosis is largely defined by clinical guidelines, using the Doppler based hemodynamic variables calculated on echocardiography, namely peak AV trans-valvular velocity, mean trans-valvular pressure gradient (mean gradient) and AV area. The AV area is calculated using the continuity equation, which encompasses both valve and LV outflow tract velocities, as well as the LV outflow tract area.

Echocardiography can also provide detailed assessment of LV geometry and function. In particular, it can assess LV hypertrophy, using the LV end-diastolic measurement of the basal posterior and septal diastolic wall thicknesses on a parasternal long axis view.

Cardiac Magnetic Resonance

Cardiac magnetic resonance (CMR) provides gold-standard measurements of LV mass, volume and ejection fraction (LVEF) as a result of its high spatial and temporal resolution. It also provides detailed views of the AV and is able to identify anatomical variants such as congenitally bicuspid valves. This is particular valuable in patients with poor acoustic windows, prohibiting adequate assessment by echocardiography (Fig. 5.4).

Cardiac magnetic resonance is able to assess potentially more sensitive measures of left ventricular dysfunction. Although reduced LVEF is strongly associated with a poor prognosis in patients with AS, this is a late finding and is preceded by impairment of diastolic function, longitudinal strain and longitudinal systolic function (subendocardial myocardial fibres oriented in a longitudinal direction are affected first by pressure overload). Longitudinal systolic function can be measured using CMR by assessing the mitral valve annular excursion between systole and diastole [16]. In addition, CMR is able to assess regional and global myocardial strain, using techniques such as myocardial tissue tagging, velocity encoding or tagged cine displacement encoding with simulated echoes (DENSE) [17].

Although pressure overloaded states such as hypertension and AS induce concentric LV remodeling and hypertrophy, several studies using CMR have suggested that asymmetric phenotypes (defined as left ventricular wall thickness >1.5 times the opposing segment) are present in up to 25% of patients [18]. While the exact mechanism is unknown, it is possible that increased wall stress could exacerbate a pre-existing genetic tendency towards a hypertrophic cardiomyopathy phenotype. Regardless, LV mass is most accurately calculated using CMR where the entire volumetric data of the LV is quantified.

There is also significant heterogeneity in the range of the LV hypertrophic response, which individual patients develop for a given severity of valve stenosis. Several studies have shown a poor correlation between the degree of LV hypertrophy and the severity of valvular stenosis (as assessed on echocardiography using aortic valve area, peak or mean gradient) [18–20]. This variation is partly explained by sex differences and clinical factors such as co-existent hypertension, age, obesity, metabolic syndrome and polymorphisms in the angiotensin-converting enzyme

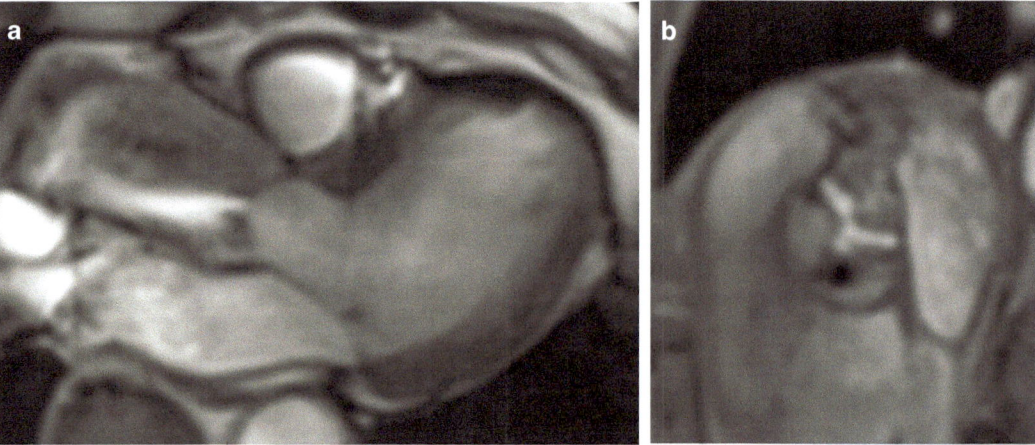

Fig. 5.4 Cardiac magnetic resonance imaging in a patient with moderate aortic stenosis. Three-chamber (**a**) and short axis (**b**) views of a patient with moderate aortic stenosis of a tri-leaflet valve

gene. Importantly, LV mass index whether calculated using echocardiography or CMR is an independent predictor of adverse cardiovascular events or all-cause mortality [18, 21, 22]. This emphasizes the importance to assess both the valve and myocardium independently.

Importantly, CMR provides a crucial advantage over other imaging techniques in that it offers assessment of myocardial fibrosis. The gold-standard assessment of fibrosis is invasive endomyocardial biopsy but this is susceptible to sampling error and associated with a small but significant risk of complications [23]. Cardiac magnetic resonance can non-invasively detect and quantify whole-heart myocardial fibrosis, using two methods, the late gadolinium enhancement (LGE), which detects replacement fibrosis and T1 mapping for diffuse fibrosis.

Late Gadolinium Enhancement

The late gadolinium enhancement (LGE) technique has been used since 1999. This method uses T1-weighted imaging sequences, 15–20 min following an intravenous bolus of gadolinium-based contrast agent. Gadolinium is too large to cross cell membranes and therefore distributes itself in the extracellular space where it accumulates in areas of extracellular volume expansion. A qualitative difference can be appreciated between "nulled" normal myocardium and areas of extracellular matrix expansion, as seen in focal replacement fibrosis, which are bright on T1-weighted sequences. These focal areas of replacement fibrosis are likely a consequence of increased coronary flow resistance in the regions of left ventricular hypertrophy and tend to occur in a mid-wall distribution [24]. This can usually be differentiated from myocardial infarction, which is another common cause of focal replacement fibrosis that characteristically occurs in a subendocardial distribution.

Mid-wall replacement fibrosis is detectable on CMR in 29–62% of patients with AS [25–27] depending on the population studied. Subendocardial LGE, suggesting previous myocardial infarction, is also commonly seen in patients with AS (10–28% [26]) as patients are often elderly with vascular risk factors and, therefore, have co-existent ischemic heart disease. Interestingly, the presence of mid-wall LGE appears more closely related to the degree of left ventricular hypertrophy rather than the severity of valve narrowing. Importantly, several studies have shown no regression in replacement fibrosis following relief of LV pressure overload associated with AV replacement [12, 28, 29], suggesting that this type of fibrosis is irreversible. As well as being a potential substrate for re-entrant arrhythmias, mid-wall fibrosis also correlates with myocardial injury as measured by high-sensitivity cardiac troponin I [30] and predicts functional recovery following surgery. Perhaps most importantly, the presence of mid-wall fibrosis has been shown to be a strong independent predictor of all–cause mortality in three separate studies [12, 26, 27], underlining its utility as an objective marker of LV decompensation in AS.

Late gadolinium enhancement techniques are unable to detect diffuse fibrosis as there is no normal myocardium present to provide visual contrast. Therefore, a considerable interest exists in the use of T1 mapping CMR assessment of diffuse fibrosis to detect and quantify fibrosis burden in AS patients (Fig. 5.5). This may potentially identify the optimal time-point to perform AV intervention before the development of irreversible pressure overload-induced pathological changes to the LV.

T1 Mapping

T1 mapping technique enables the detection and quantification of diffuse myocardial fibrosis, an earlier form of myocardial fibrosis. This process is characterised by collagen deposition and associated expansion of the extracellular volume (ECV), which precedes replacement fibrosis. This progressive change occurs due to an increased requirement for extracellular matrix to support the hypertrophied myocytes as a consequence of an increased LV afterload, triggering increased myofibroblast collagen synthesis.

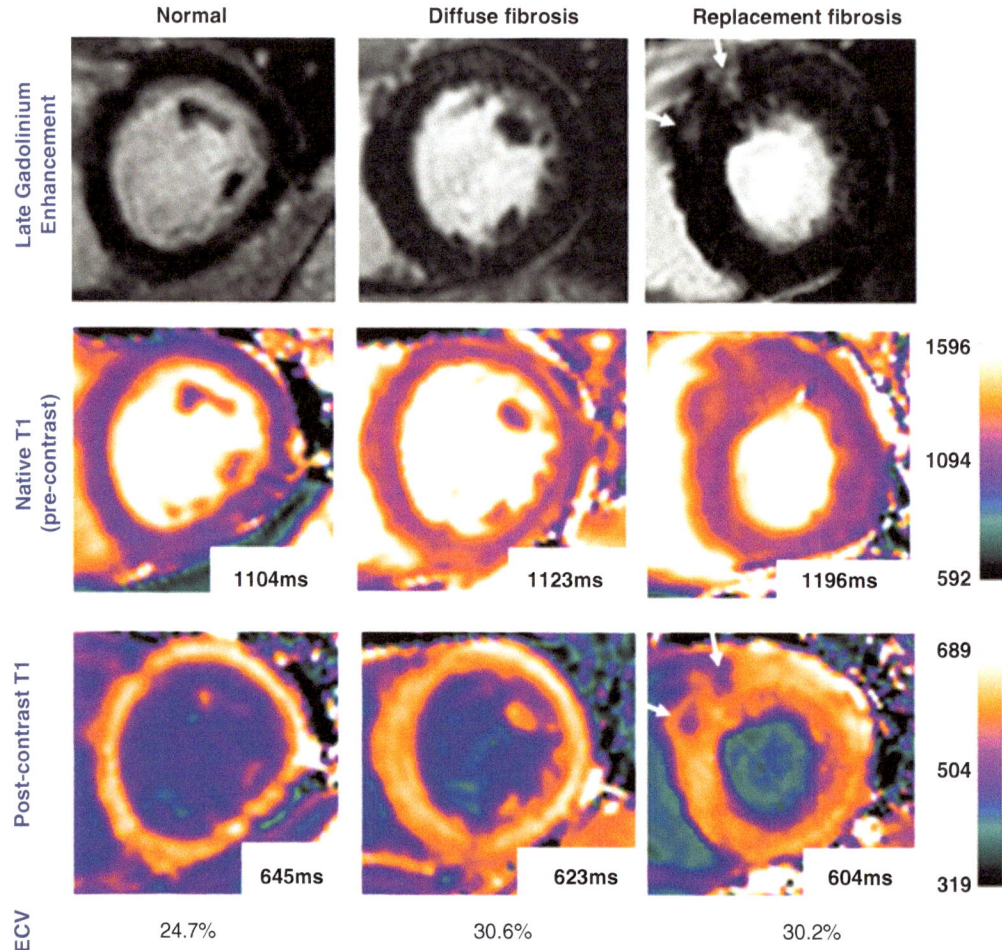

Fig. 5.5 T1 mapping and late gadolinium enhancement in aortic stenosis. Left column: a healthy control patient with normal myocardium, extracellular volume values and no late gadolinium enhancement. Middle column: a patient with severe aortic stenosis with raised extracellular volume indicating diffuse fibrosis. Right column: a patient with severe aortic stenosis with asymmetrical anteroseptal left ventricular hypertrophy, a raised extracellular volume and mid-wall late gadolinium enhancement (white arrows)

As described in the earlier chapters, there are a variety of T1 mapping measures that have been studied in literature. The evidence for and utility of each of these measurements in the assessment of patients with AS will be examined in detail.

Native T1

The use of native T1 has many advantages. It has good reproducibility in some studies involving patients with AS [31]. Scanning times are shorter than the equivalent contrast-based approaches.

Indeed, the lack of gadolinium-based contrast agents makes this approach particularly attractive in patients with advanced renal impairment (EGFR <30 mL/min/1.73 m^2) and other contraindications to contrast.

Native T1 values are influenced by the changes in the molecular composition or water content in any of the tissue compartments of imaged tissue. In some conditions such as the hypertrophic cardiomyopathy, the most significant changes are intracellular abnormality with sarcomeric and myocyte disarray. Much of the current literature regarding AS focuses on the extracellular compartment where extracellular matrix expansion with collagen deposition (myocardial fibrosis) causes an increase in native T1 values. Other conditions show similar increases in native T1 due to deposition of other proteins, such as in amyloidosis. However, water content, whether intra or extravascular, is an important determinant of native T1. For example, patients with myocarditis have raised native T1 values in areas of myocardial inflammation due to the presence of myocardial edema. The intravascular compartment is often overlooked as highlighted in a recent study using adenosine stress CMR. Patients with severe AS have increased resting coronary flow volume and reduced flow reserve [32]. Native T1 values also increase with vasodilator pharmacological stress, presumably due to increased water volume in in the imaged tissue associated with increased myocardial blood flow. This may partially explain why native T1 values are higher in patients with aortic stenosis (with increased resting coronary flow volume) compared to controls but both increase to a similar level at pharmacological stress [28].

In general, native T1 has demonstrated a good correlation with diffuse myocardial fibrosis on histological analysis [33–35] although this has not been a universal finding [36]. Moreover, histology is performed on biopsy samples obtained at the time of AV replacement. This approach is, therefore, restricted to patients with severe symptomatic disease. The T1 mapping data in less advanced stages of the disease have not been histologically validated.

Bull and colleagues first investigated the use of native T1 in 109 patients with moderate or severe aortic stenosis. Native T1 values were raised in patients with aortic stenosis compared to 33 age and sex matched controls. Both AV area and LV mass index were independently associated with native T1 values [33]. Several other studies have shown that native T1 is able to differentiate patients with AS from controls albeit with considerable overlap in values between the two groups [31, 37]. Chin and colleagues investigated various T1 mapping measures at 3 tesla (3T) in 20 patients with AS and 20 healthy volunteers. While native T1 had excellent intra and

inter–observer variability and acceptable scan-rescan reproducibility, it was unable to discriminate between AS and control subjects [37]. This finding may have been due to a wider spectrum of AS severity in this study (mild to severe) compared to the previous studies, which involved patients with more severe disease.

The accumulation of diffuse myocardial fibrosis leads to progressive impairment in LV function. Although no studies have yet shown a link between native T1 and reduced ejection fraction in aortic stenosis, native T1 has been associated with these earlier measures of left ventricular dysfunction. Lee and colleagues assessed 80 asymptomatic patients with moderate or severe aortic stenosis using 3T cardiac magnetic resonance and included echocardiographic speckle tracking imaging. Native T1 values showed a good correlation with measures of impaired global longitudinal strain and diastolic dysfunction (mean e' and left atrial volume) [34].

The primary utility of native T1 in clinical practice will be to establish normal native T1 values in healthy hearts and, therefore, to define cut-off values of abnormal levels of fibrosis in cardiac pathology. To date, two studies have attempted to do this in patients with AS. Lee and colleagues showed that at 3T, a cut off of 1190 ms could discriminate between moderate and severe AS with c-statistic of 0.704 [34]. However, given the poor correlation between AS severity and the LV remodeling response, it may be more useful to identify native T1 cut-offs that predict future adverse events. In another recent study of 40 patients undergoing AV replacement (AS 77.5% and aortic regurgitation 15%) or root replacement (7.5%) with concurrent myocardial biopsies, Kockova and colleagues defined an optimum native T1 cut-off value of 1010 ms, generating a sensitivity of 90%, specificity of 73% and c-statistic of 0.82 to detect severe diffuse fibrosis on histology (defined as collagen volume fraction of >30%) [35]. Again, outcome studies are needed to show that these cut-offs can detect patients at higher risk of future adverse events.

The major limitation of native T1 is that the values obtained are specific to the sequence, scanner and magnetic field strength. As such, a reliable comparison between the clinical centers is challenging and has limited the guideline for reference ranges to define health and disease states, which in turn limits clinical applicability.

Post-contrast T1 and the Partition Coefficient

Intravenous gadolinium shortens the T1 values and localizes the extracellular space. These behaviours can be utilized in conjunction with T1 mapping to aid further in the assessment of diffuse myocardial fibrosis. The use of equilibrium CMR (where a constant intravenous gadolinium-based contrast media infusion is used to create contrast equilibrium) have been supplanted by dynamic equilibrium techniques (where imaging is performed at a set time following bolus administration when it is assumed to be a dynamic equilibrium between myocardial and blood gadolinium concentrations). However, the isolated post-contrast T1 values are highly dependent on an individual's gadolinium kinetics and the varying time to image post contrast administration results in poor scan-rescan reproducibility, limiting its clinical use [37].

Correction to post-contrast T1 values can be performed by calculating the partition coefficient (λ), which calculates the ratio of myocardial T1 to blood T1 and corrects for the variation caused by an individual's gadolinium contrast kinetics. It has a much improved scan-rescan variability compared to the isolated post-contrast T1 and differentiates AS from control subjects [37].

Extracellular Volume Fraction

The further use of the hematocrit to calculate the blood volume in turn allows the myocardial volume to be estimated (assuming contrast equilibrium between these two compartments). As gadolinium is purely extracellular, its distribution in the myocardial volume is equal to the extracellular volume (ECV) and this measure is termed ECV fraction. Although the extracellular space contains not just collagen but other extracellular matrix components, including myocardial capillaries, the ECV measure has been shown to correlate well with histological collagen volume fraction on myocardial biopsy samples in multiple studies of AS patients undergoing AV replacement [35, 38–40].

Extracellular volume was first validated in AS in 2010 by Flett and colleagues who used equilibrium contrast CMR at 1.5T to investigate 18 patients with severe AS who underwent myocardial biopsy at the time of AV replacement. Extracellular volume strongly correlated ($r^2 = 0.86$) with collagen volume fraction as assessed by picrosirius red quantification on histology [39]. Equilibrium contrast CMR involved a highly complex protocol, requiring an extra 30–90 min of patient time in the radiology department.

Flett and colleagues went on to examine, using similar methods in 63 patients with severe AS undergoing AV replacement and 30 healthy controls [14]. Diffuse myocardial fibrosis was estimated using a line of best fit correlation between histological fibrosis (collagen volume fraction) and CMR obtained ECV values from their previous study [39]. Patients with AS had more diffuse myocardial fibrosis compared to control subjects (18 versus 13%) although these values overlapped significantly. Diffuse fibrosis was associated with diastolic dysfunction and impaired functional status as measured by 6-min walk test independent of age, sex, LVEF, AV area and presence of LGE [14].

Extracellular volume has excellent reproducibility and appears to have superior inter-observer, intra-observer and scan-rescan reproducibility compared to other T1 measures at 3T [37]. This study used simplified dynamic equilibrium sequences using a contrast bolus injection with imaging performed 10–20 min post administration, which have been shown to give comparable results to the more complex equilibrium contrast infusion techniques. These bolus techniques have, therefore, almost universally been adopted. Extracellular volume was also found to be significantly greater in patients with AS compared to healthy controls although a large degree of overlap was observed. Similar findings have been observed in other studies [14, 41]; however, the control populations in these studies were younger and common co-morbidities such as hypertension or diabetes were excluded. In a recent study, extracellular volume was unable to differentiate between patients with asymptomatic moderate or severe aortic stenosis in age, gender and co-morbidity matched controls; nevertheless, these studies were most likely under-powered [31].

As with the native T1, establishing the normal range of ECV values in healthy controls and disease specific cut-offs is essential for clinical utility. Extracellular volume is less dependent on scanning sequence and magnetic field strength but some variability remains [38]. As detailed above, Kockova and colleagues examined 40 patients (77.5% with severe aortic stenosis) who underwent AV replacement and myocardial biopsy. They showed that a cut-off ECV of ≥0.32 was able to detect severe myocardial fibrosis (defined as >30% by histology) with a sensitivity of 80%, specificity of 90% and c-statistic of 0.85. The clinical utility of this cut-off and long-term prognostic value are unknown. Defining the clinically relevant cut-off values remains key. Overall, a higher ECV has been shown to be predictive of all-cause mortality and heart failure admissions in heterogeneous populations with cardiac disease (excluding hypertrophic cardiomyopathy and amyloidosis) [42, 43]; however, this has not been examined in an aortic stenosis population to date.

Absolute Extracellular Volume

The limitation of current T1 measurement is that they universally show a substantial overlap between AS patients and healthy controls, limiting their clinical application. Although ECV is conceptually a particularly attractive measure, it assesses diffuse fibrosis as a percentage of the left ventricular myocardial volume and, therefore, a measure of relative fibrosis. Compared to other myocardial pathology, this may be of less use in AS which is characterised by a reactive increase in both LV mass and diffuse myocardial fibrosis in response to sustained pressure over-

load. As such, the relative fibrosis may not change as disease progresses. An absolute measure of whole heart fibrosis, such as the absolute extracellular volume (extracellular volume x end-diastolic myocardial volume) may therefore be more useful in staging disease and tracking changes in fibrosis over time.

The use of extracellular volume indexed to body surface area (indexed extracellular volume, iECV) was examined in 166 patients with AS of whom approximately half had severe aortic stenosis. Normal levels of iECV were defined in 37 age and sex matched controls (normal iECV <22.5 mL/m^2). Patient classification by the presence of abnormal diffuse fibrosis (iECV >22.5 mL/m^2) or replacement fibrosis (mid-wall late gadolinium enhancement) showed a stepwise progression in troponin I concentration, diastolic dysfunction and longitudinal systolic dysfunction from patients with no fibrosis to diffuse and then to replacement fibrosis, which was also associated with unadjusted all-cause mortality [44]. Further longitudinal studies are necessary but this seems to be a very promising approach to address some of the issues of disease discrimination.

Barriers to Widespread Adoption

Cardiac magnetic resonance is an expensive technology and although there has been an expansion of capacity over recent years, access is still limited with considerable geographical variation [45]. A major limitation of current T1 mapping techniques is the overlap in the values between patients with AS and healthy controls. Further work is needed to select the most useful T1 measure and acquisition sequence to optimise the prognostic capability. T1 values differ depending on CMR scanner, sequence and magnetic field strength, which hinder collaboration between research centers, delay the determination of normal reference ranges, and confound the healthy and diseased states. Although such normal reference range has been described that are scanner and sequence specific [46], a major challenge remains in standardizing the techniques, identifying the widely applicable reference range, and establishing the prognostically significant cut-off values for T1 measurements, which represent clinically relevant applications for myocardial fibrosis.

Potential Uses of T1 Mapping

T1 mapping measurements may find a role as surrogate end-points in clinical trials. Native T1 and ECV are currently well validated against histology for the presence of myocardial fibrosis and the use of these measures as surrogate end-points may allow easier testing of novel therapies or management strategies for AS with greater statistical power, requiring smaller numbers of patients.

T1 mapping assessment may be able to refine decision making regarding AV intervention. The risks associated with surgical AV replacement have been falling for decades due to improved surgical technology and peri-operative care. In addition, the introduction of percutaneous transcatheter aortic valve replacement (TAVR) procedures for high-risk or inoperable patients has enabled AV replacement at relatively low risk with good short to medium term outcomes [47, 48]. A recent trial showed encouraging outcomes using TAVR in intermediate risk patients [49] and it seems likely that TAVR will see huge expansion in coming years. With lower risk options available for treating severe AS, the risk–benefit balance may move in favour of intervention earlier in the disease process as the potential benefits from valve intervention will outweigh the small risks of intervention. The use of T1 mapping to assess diffuse fibrosis burden may become a method to identify high risk asymptomatic patients who will benefit from these percutaneous or minimally invasive AV interventions.

Future Directions

T1 mapping in AS is an exciting and rapidly progressing field. For example, novel contrast agents are in development that could allow non-invasive assessment of extracellular matrix composition.

Gadolinium-based collagen and elastin specific contrast agents bind to collagen and tropoelastin respectively in pre-clinical mouse models, and have a longer washout period from the myocardium increasing the contrast-to-noise ratio on delayed cardiac magnetic resonance sequences [50, 51]. Increased tropoelastin synthesis is associated with improved ejection fraction in mouse models of myocardial infarction and both of these agents could potentially monitor the effects of novel therapies in the future. Further studies using these agents are pending.

Techniques to assess T1 measurements are also evolving. Although the use of bolus administration of gadolinium-based contrast agent has simplified the technique compared to previous equilibrium contrast CMR, novel methods to reduce the complexity and duration of the scan would be advantageous. In particular, Treibel and colleagues have shown that it may be possible to calculate a so called "synthetic extracellular volume" based on the linear relationship between blood relaxivity (1/T1) and the hematocrit. This would simplify the technique by removing the need for hematocrit sampling [43].

There is also interest in the use of CMR to assess valve leaflet composition, given the excellent spatial resolution and exquisite tissue characterization. Preliminary *ex vivo* work with explanted AV leaflets showed that CMR displayed excellent sensitivity and specificity for the identification of both mineralization and fibrosis with lower accuracy for lipid-rich tissues [52]. However, clinical applications are limited at present as CMR currently lacks the temporal resolution to perform such imaging *in vivo* due to valve leaflet motion.

Conclusion

The importance of the myocardial response to progressive AS is increasingly recognized. Cardiac magnetic resonance offers gold-standard measurements of LV volumes and mass while also providing whole heart quantification of diffuse and replacement myocardial fibrosis. These findings may be linked to adverse outcomes. The use of T1 mapping to identify early LV decompensation may allow intervention to relieve pressure overload before the onset of irreversible LV dysfunction. The challenge is now to refine T1 mapping techniques to determine the normal reference range and establish their prognostic significance. We await the results of randomised clinical trials that demonstrate the benefit of management strategies involving T1 mapping measurements.

References

1. Iung B, Baron G, Butchart EG, Delahaye F, Gohlke-Bärwolf C, Levang OW, et al. A prospective survey of patients with valvular heart disease in Europe: the Euro Heart Survey on Valvular Heart Disease. Eur Heart J. 2003;24(13):1231–43.
2. Nkomo VT, Gardin JM, Skelton TN, Gottdiener JS, Scott CG, Enriquez-Sarano M. Burden of valvular heart diseases: a population-based study. Lancet. 2006;368(9540):1005–11.
3. Ross J, Braunwald E. Aortic stenosis. Circulation. 1968;38(1 Suppl):61–7.
4. Connolly HM, Oh JK, Orszulak TA, Osborn SL, Roger VL, Hodge DO, et al. Aortic valve replacement for aortic stenosis with severe left ventricular dysfunction. Prognostic indicators. Circulation. 1997;95(10):2395–400.
5. Tribouilloy C, Levy F, Rusinaru D, Guéret P, Petit-Eisenmann H, Baleynaud S, et al. Outcome after aortic valve replacement for low-flow/low-gradient aortic stenosis without contractile reserve on dobutamine stress echocardiography. J Am Coll Cardiol. 2009;53(20):1865–73.
6. Dweck MR, Boon NA, Newby DE. Calcific aortic stenosis: a disease of the valve and the myocardium. J Am Coll Cardiol. 2012;60(19):1854–63.
7. Dweck MR, Jones C, Joshi NV, Fletcher AM, Richardson H, White A, et al. Assessment of valvular calcification and inflammation by positron emission tomography in patients with aortic stenosis. Circulation. 2012;125(1):76–86.
8. Rossebø AB, Pedersen TR, Boman K, Brudi P, Chambers JB, Egstrup K, et al. Intensive lipid lowering with simvastatin and ezetimibe in aortic stenosis. N Engl J Med. 2008;359(13):1343–56.
9. Cowell SJ, Newby DE, Prescott RJ, Bloomfield P, Reid J, Northridge DB, et al. A randomized trial of intensive lipid-lowering therapy in calcific aortic stenosis. N Engl J Med. 2005;352(23):2389–97.
10. Chan KL, Teo K, Dumesnil JG, Ni A, Tam J, Investigators A. Effect of lipid lowering with rosuvastatin on progression of aortic stenosis results of the aortic stenosis progression observation: measuring effects of rosuvastatin (ASTRONOMER) trial. Circulation. 2010;121(2):306–U247.
11. Hein S, Arnon E, Kostin S, Schönburg M, Elsässer A, Polyakova V, et al. Progression from compensated hypertrophy to failure in the pressure-overloaded human heart: structural deterioration and compensatory mechanisms. Circulation. 2003;107(7):984–91.
12. Azevedo CF, Nigri M, Higuchi ML, Pomerantzeff PM, Spina GS, Sampaio RO, et al. Prognostic significance of myocardial fibrosis quantification by histopathology and magnetic resonance imaging in patients with severe aortic valve disease. J Am Coll Cardiol. 2010;56(4):278–87.
13. Krayenbeuhl HP, Hess OM, Monrad ES, Schneider J, Mall G, Turina M. Left-ventricular myocardial structure in aortic-valve disease before, intermediate, and late after aortic-valve replacement. Circulation. 1989;79(4):744–55.
14. Flett AS, Sado DM, Quarta G, Mirabel M, Pellerin D, Herrey AS, et al. Diffuse myocardial fibrosis in severe aortic stenosis: an equilibrium contrast cardiovascular magnetic resonance study. Eur Heart J Cardiovasc Imaging. 2012;13(10):jes102–826.
15. Shah ASV, Chin CWL, Vassiliou V, Cowell SJ, Doris M, Kwok TC, et al. Left ventricular hypertrophy with strain and aortic stenosis. Circulation. 2014;130(18):1607–16.
16. Dobson LE, Musa TA, Fairbairn TA, Uddin A, Blackman DJ, Ripley DP, et al. CMR assessment of longitudinal left ventricular function following transcatheter aortic valve implantation (TAVI) for severe aortic stenosis. J Cardiovasc Magn Reson. 2015;17(1):P180.
17. Ibrahim E-SH. Myocardial tagging by cardiovascular magnetic resonance: evolution of techniques—pulse sequences, analysis algorithms, and applications. J Cardiovasc Magn Reson. 2011;13(1):36.
18. Dweck MR, Joshi S, Murigu T, Gulati A, Alpendurada F, Jabbour A, et al. Left ventricular remodeling and hypertrophy in patients with aortic stenosis: insights from cardiovascular magnetic resonance. J Cardiovasc Magn Reson. 2012;14(1):1–1.
19. Gunther S, Grossman W. Determinants of ventricular function in pressure-overload hypertrophy in man. Circulation. 1979;59(4):679–88.
20. Salcedo EE, Korzick DH, Currie PJ, Stewart WJ, Lever HM, Goormastic M. Determinants of left ventricular hypertrophy in patients with aortic stenosis. Cleve Clin J Med. 1989;56(6):590–6.
21. Cioffi G, Faggiano P, Vizzardi E, Tarantini L, Cramariuc D, Gerdts E, et al. Prognostic effect of inappropriately high left ventricular mass in asymptomatic severe aortic stenosis. Heart. 2011;97(4):301–7.
22. Gerdts E, Rossebø AB, Pedersen TR, Cioffi G, Lønnebakken MT, Cramariuc D, et al. Relation of left ventricular mass to prognosis in initially asymptomatic mild to moderate aortic valve stenosis. Circ Cardiovasc Imaging. 2015;8(11):e003644; discussion e003644.
23. Yilmaz A, Kindermann I, Kindermann M, Mahfoud F, Ukena C, Athanasiadis A, et al. Comparative evaluation of left and right ventricular endomyocardial biopsy: differences in complication rate and diagnostic performance. Circulation. 2010;122(9):900–9.

24. Debl K, Djavidani B, Buchner S, Lipke C, Nitz W, Feuerbach S, et al. Delayed hyperenhancement in magnetic resonance imaging of left ventricular hypertrophy caused by aortic stenosis and hypertrophic cardiomyopathy: visualisation of focal fibrosis. Heart. 2006;92(10):1447–51.

25. Rudolph A, Abdel-Aty H, Bohl S, Boyé P, Zagrosek A, Dietz R, et al. Noninvasive detection of fibrosis applying contrast-enhanced cardiac magnetic resonance in different forms of left ventricular hypertrophy relation to remodeling. J Am Coll Cardiol. 2009;53(3):284–91.

26. Dweck MR, Joshi S, Murigu T, Alpendurada F, Jabbour A, Melina G, et al. Midwall fibrosis is an independent predictor of mortality in patients with aortic stenosis. J Am Coll Cardiol. 2011;58(12):1271–9.

27. Barone-Rochette G, Piérard S, De Meester de Ravenstein C, Seldrum S, Melchior J, Maes F, et al. Prognostic significance of LGE by CMR in aortic stenosis patients undergoing valve replacement. J Am Coll Cardiol. 2014;64(2):144–54.

28. Mahmod M, Piechnik SK, Levelt E, Ferreira VM, Francis JM, Lewis A, et al. Adenosine stress native T1 mapping in severe aortic stenosis: evidence for a role of the intravascular compartment on myocardial T1 values. J Cardiovasc Magn Reson. 2014;16(1):92.

29. Weidemann F, Herrmann S, Störk S, Niemann M, Frantz S, Lange V, et al. Impact of myocardial fibrosis in patients with symptomatic severe aortic stenosis. Circulation. 2009;120(7):577–84.

30. Chin CWL, Shah ASV, McAllister DA, Joanna Cowell S, Alam S, Langrish JP, et al. High-sensitivity troponin I concentrations are a marker of an advanced hypertrophic response and adverse outcomes in patients with aortic stenosis. Eur Heart J. 2014;35(34):2312–21.

31. Singh A, Horsfield MA, Bekele S, Khan JN, Greiser A, McCann GP. Myocardial T1 and extracellular volume fraction measurement in asymptomatic patients with aortic stenosis: reproducibility and comparison with age-matched controls. Eur Heart J Cardiovasc Imaging. 2015;16(7):763–70.

32. Eberli FR, Ritter M, Schwitter J, Bortone A, Schneider J, Hess OM, et al. Coronary reserve in patients with aortic valve disease before and after successful aortic valve replacement. Eur Heart J. 1991;12(2):127–38.

33. Bull S, White SK, Piechnik SK, Flett AS, Ferreira VM, Loudon M, et al. Human non-contrast T1 values and correlation with histology in diffuse fibrosis. Heart. 2013;99(13):932–7.

34. Lee S-P, Lee W, Lee JM, Park E-A, Kim H-K, Kim Y-J, et al. Assessment of diffuse myocardial fibrosis by using MR imaging in asymptomatic patients with aortic stenosis. Radiology. 2015;274(2):359–69.

35. Kockova R, Kacer P, Pirk J, Maly J, Sukupova L, Sikula V, et al. Native T1 relaxation time and extracellular volume fraction as accurate markers of diffuse myocardial fibrosis in heart valve disease—comparison with targeted left ventricular myocardial biopsy. Circ J. 2016;80(5):1202–9.

36. De Meester de Ravenstein C, Bouzin C, Lazam S, Boulif J, Amzulescu M, Melchior J, et al. Histological validation of measurement of diffuse interstitial myocardial fibrosis by myocardial extravascular volume fraction from Modified Look-Locker imaging (MOLLI) T1 mapping at 3 T. J Cardiovasc Magn Reson. 2015;17(1):48.

37. Chin CWL, Semple S, Malley T, White AC, Mirsadraee S, Weale PJ, et al. Optimization and comparison of myocardial T1 techniques at 3T in patients with aortic stenosis. Eur Heart J Cardiovasc Imaging. 2014;15(5):556–65.

38. Fontana M, White SK, Banypersad SM. Comparison of T1 mapping techniques for ECV quantification. Histological validation and reproducibility of ShMOLLI versus multibreath-hold T1 quantification equilibrium contrast CMR. J Cardiovasc Magn Reson. 2012;14:88.

39. Flett AS, Hayward MP, Ashworth MT, Hansen MS, Taylor AM, Elliott PM, et al. Equilibrium contrast cardiovascular magnetic resonance for the measurement of diffuse myocardial fibrosis: preliminary validation in humans. Circulation. 2010;122(2):138–44.

40. White SK, Sado DM, Fontana M, Banypersad SM, Maestrini V, Flett AS, et al. T1 mapping for myocardial extracellular volume measurement by CMR: bolus only versus primed infusion technique. JACC Cardiovasc Imaging. 2013;6(9):955–62.

41. Sado DM, Flett AS, Banypersad SM, White SK, Maestrini V, Quarta G, et al. Cardiovascular magnetic resonance measurement of myocardial extracellular volume in health and disease. Heart. 2012;98(19):1436–41.

42. Wong TC, Piehler K, Meier CG, Testa SM, Klock AM, Aneizi AA, et al. Association between extracellular matrix expansion quantified by cardiovascular magnetic resonance and short term mortality. Circulation. 2012;126(10):1206–16.

43. Treibel TA, Fontana M, Maestrini V, Castelletti S, Rosmini S, Simpson J, et al. Automatic Measurement of the Myocardial Interstitium: synthetic extracellular volume quantification without hematocrit sampling. JACC Cardiovasc Imaging. 2016;9(1):54–63.

44. https://www.ncbi.nlm.nih.gov/pubmed/28017384.

45. Antony R, Daghem M, McCann GP, Daghem S, Moon J, Pennell DJ, et al. Cardiovascular magnetic resonance activity in the United Kingdom: a survey on behalf of the British Society of Cardiovascular Magnetic Resonance. J Cardiovasc Magn Reson. 2011;13(1):57.

46. Dabir D, Child N, Kalra A, Rogers T, Gebker R, Jabbour A, et al. Reference values for healthy human myocardium using a T1 mapping methodology: results from the International T1 Multicenter cardiovascular magnetic resonance study. J Cardiovasc Magn Reson. 2014;16(1):69.

47. Mack MJ, Leon MB, Smith CR, Miller DC, Moses JW, Tuzcu EM, et al. 5-year outcomes of transcatheter aortic valve replacement or surgical aortic valve replacement for high surgical risk patients with aortic stenosis (PARTNER 1): a randomised controlled trial. Lancet. 2015;385(9986):2477–84.

48. Kapadia SR, Leon MB, Makkar RR, Tuzcu EM, Svensson LG, Kodali S, et al. 5-year outcomes of transcatheter aortic valve replacement compared with standard treatment for patients with inoperable aortic stenosis (PARTNER 1): a randomised controlled trial. Lancet. 2015;385(9986):2485–91.

49. Leon MB, Smith CR, Mack MJ, Makkar RR, Svensson LG, Kodali SK, et al. Transcatheter or surgical aortic-valve replacement in intermediate-risk patients. N Engl J Med. 2016;374(17):1609–20.

50. Helm PA, Caravan P, French BA, Jacques V, Shen L, Xu Y, et al. Postinfarction myocardial scar-ring in mice: molecular MR imaging with use of a collagen-targeting contrast agent. Radiology. 2008;247(3):788–96.

51. Wildgruber M, Bielicki I, Aichler M, Kosanke K, Feuchtinger A, Settles M, et al. Assessment of myocardial infarction and postinfarction scar remodeling with an elastin-specific magnetic resonance agent. Circ Cardiovasc Imaging. 2014;7(2):321–9.

52. Ven Le F, Tizón-Marcos H, Fuchs C, Mathieu P, Pibarot P, Larose E. Valve tissue characterization by magnetic resonance imaging in calcific aortic valve disease. Can J Cardiol. 2014;30(12):1676–83.

T1 Mapping in Peri-infarct Injury in Ischemic Cardiomyopathy

Yuko Tada and Rajesh Dash

Ischemic Cardiomyopathy and T1 Mapping

Despite advances in post-myocardial infarction (post-MI) care, sudden death remains a major risk within the first 30 days of a myocardial infarction [1, 2]. As a result, there is unique clinical value in understanding whether a patient possesses significant amounts of a 'mixed injury' in the peri-infarction region (PIR) in ischemic cardiomyopathy. This PIR region has been linked to arrhythmogenicity and, therefore, sudden cardiac death in post-MI patients [3]. Because the PIR is typically of variable viability (a mixture of live and dead cells as well as fibrosis), there are technical challenges to identifying and quantifying PIR volume and the degree of heterogeneous composition using non-invasive imaging techniques. Recently, cardiac MRI, which has both the tissue characterization abilities and spatiotemporal resolution to both localize and accurately quantify these regions, has shown promising and innovative inroads into

this measurement. T1 mapping, using multiple contrast agents, affords the ability to not only discriminate the presence and amount of PIR, but to also grade the degree of 'variable viability' within the PIR, all of which may correlate with both salvageable myocardium as well as arrhythmogenic potential [4]. This chapter will review the advances in T1 mapping in ischemic cardiomyopathy.

T1 Mapping Techniques in Ischemic Cardiomyopathy

Advances in T1 sequences in cardiac MRI have enabled more rapid acquisition and high-resolution mapping of the T1 maps of the myocardium to denote more subtle levels of either cellular death/injury when using gadolinium-based contrast agents. Conversely, the recent use of a manganese-based contrast agent has been optimized to reveal the extent of myocardial cell viability, opening the door to specific questions that dictate one's approach to CMR T1 imaging of the myocardium. Both contrast agents, with unique strengths and limitations, contribute to our understanding of the role of the PIR in clinical management of ischemic cardiomyopathy patients.

Y. Tada, MD, PhD
Division of Cardiovascular Medicine, Department of Medicine, Stanford University, Stanford, CA, USA
e-mail: ytada@stanford.edu

R. Dash, MD, PhD (✉)
Division of Cardiovascular Medicine, Department of Medicine, Stanford University Medical Center, Stanford, CA, USA
e-mail: rhombus@stanford.edu

© Springer International Publishing AG, part of Springer Nature 2018
P. C. Yang (ed.), *T1-Mapping in Myocardial Disease*, https://doi.org/10.1007/978-3-319-91110-6_6

Gadolinium Enhanced Delayed Enhancement

In the setting of ischemic injury to the heart, a sudden drop in myocardial blood flow (MBF) results in a low-flow state to segment(s) of the heart and a significant increase in extracellular volume in affected regions. These changes produce an accumulation of Gadolinium in those segments, which does not cross intact cell membranes but instead resides in the extracellular space, leading to a marked T1 shortening signal effect. Most of our clinical interpretation of delayed gadolinium enhancement relies upon relative signal differences between healthy (nulled) or injured/dead tissue. There has been considerable research and clinical validation of how gadolinium enhancement measurements can predict the functional recovery of infarcted segments of myocardium after revascularization [5]. Typically, a segment with less than 50% thickness enhancement and at least 5 mm of non-enhanced myocardium has a favorable chance to functionally recover upon revascularization. Indeed, the amount of enhancement as a percentage of total LV mass is not only highly predictive of cardiovascular events in ischemic cardiomyopathy patients, but is superior to ejection fraction and ventricular volumes, which have traditionally been used for such estimations (Table 6.1) [6].

Role of PIR in Predicting Cardiovascular Outcomes in Ischemic Cardiomyopathy

Building upon the predictive findings of the proportion of total myocardial mass with delayed enhancement, a study was performed using just signal intensity without formal T1 mapping [4]. This study noted that a more detailed analysis of the delayed enhancement pattern of ischemic cardiomyopathy patients was able to identify a PIR in which the size of the PIR and the variability in the signal intensity both correlated with cardiovascular outcomes (see reprinted Fig. 6.1). This study suggested that a true T1 map of the infarct region and PIR may indicate the likelihood of arrhythmogenesis on an individualized patient basis.

T1 Mapping Using Gadolinium Enhancement

Because of the T1 shortening properties of gadolinium distribution in the heart, T1 mapping of infarcted regions is a natural extension of delayed enhancement, as the true T1 value of each voxel of myocardium can be mapped from both within and immediately surrounding the infarcted tissue. This technique has been correlated with visual assessments of infarct size as well as delineation of PIR, but also generates a calculated extracellular volume (ECV) that can characterize infarct zones and PIR [7]. The advent of T1 mapping allows a more detailed PIR assessment by identifying the true T1 value of every voxel within the infarct zone and PIR. Thresholds of T1 signal for inclusion within the infarct zone or PIR then lead to more precise derivations of each region's boundaries.

Limitations to Gadolinium Enhancement

Today, gadolinium delayed enhancement MRI is used clinically as the gold standard for infarct sizing in ischemic cardiomyopathy.

Table 6.1 The proportion of non-transmural versus transmural segments of myocardial infarction, correlation with event rates

	Cardiovascular events (+)	Cardiovascular events (−)	p-value
Non-transmural MI (1–75% scar of myocardium)	18.4 ± 14.0	13.8 ± 11.2	0.049
1–25% scar of myocardium	9.2 ± 11.0	6.7 ± 9.3	0.12
26–50% scar of myocardium	9.2 ± 10.6	3.2 ± 3.6	0.03
51–75% scar of myocardium	3.5 ± 4.2	4.0 ± 4.5	0.30
Transmural MI (76–100% scar of myocardium)	5.8 ± 10.2	7.2 ± 11.4	0.28

Values are expressed as a mean ± SD

Reprinted showing the correlation of the % of enhancement of total myocardial mass with cardiovascular event rates [6]

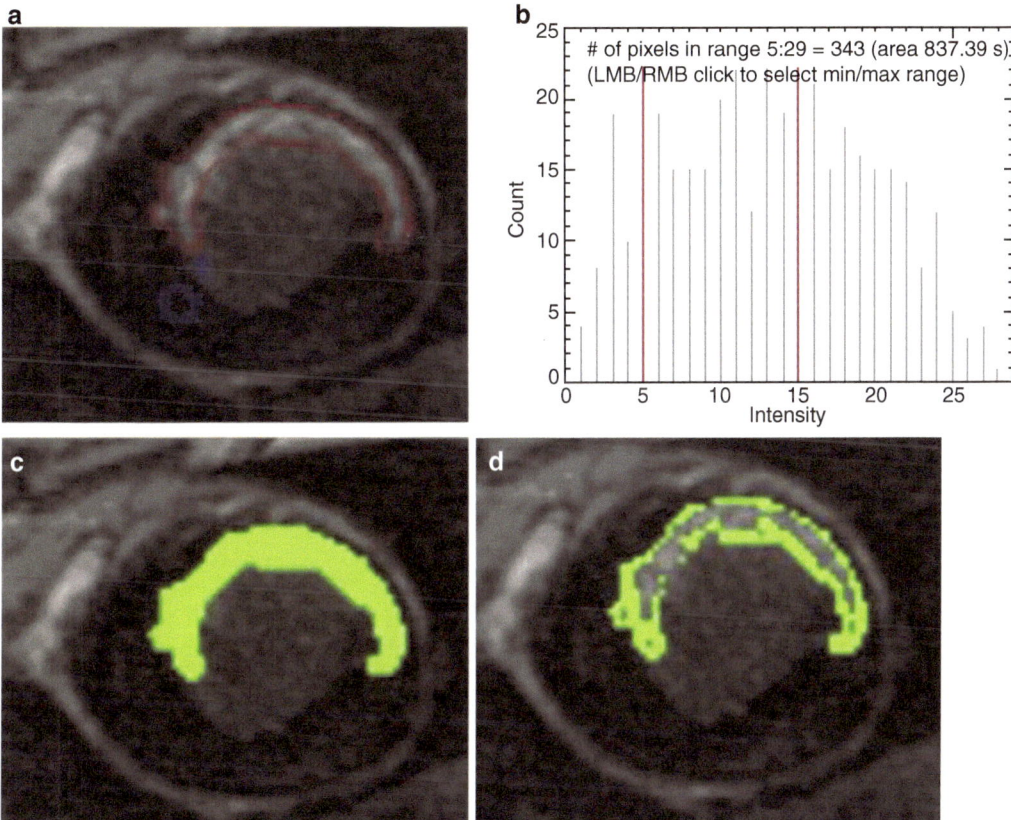

Fig. 6.1 Determining tissue heterogeneity. (**a**) An area of late gadolinium enhancement (LGE) was identified (*red*) and was planimetered by a trained observer. The observer then planimetered a region of interest (ROI) in the remote, noninfarcted myocardium (*blue*). (**b**) The maximum signal intensity (SI) within the area of LGE was determined (LGE SI max = 29). The maximum SI within the remote ROI region was determined (ROI SI max = 5). The infarct core was defined as the zone with SI >50% of the maximal SI in the infarct (SI core = 15–29), whereas the border was defined as the zone with an SI > maximum SI in the remote ROI but <50% of maximal SI of the infarct (SI border = 5–15, between the *red lines*; the value of 15 is included in the border zone). (**c**) The total scar is depicted in *green*. (**d**) The border zone is depicted in *green*. The area of the core and border zones was determined, and the tissue mass (g) was calculated by the following: area × slice thickness × 1.05. LMB = left main bronchus; RMB = right main bronchus. (Reprinted from Heidary et al. JACC Vol 55, Issue 24, 15 June 2010, 2762–2768)

However, a relative signal difference using human visual assessment is prone to insensitivity to subtle signal differences that may be present, which may represent variability between a truly 'infarcted' myocardial region versus just an 'injured' myocardial region. The reliability and precision of defining those affected regions is subject to the individual reader. Our group recently published that a gross overestimation of truly infarcted myocardial segments is likely if you rely only upon relative gadolinium update in the setting of ischemic cardiomyopathy [8]. As a result, identifying gradations of myocardial injury or viability within the penumbra or border zones or PIR of infarction may be clinically relevant when revascularization decisions are made. Moreover, if arrhythmogenesis consideration becomes a future consideration for medical or defibrillator management of ischemic cardiomyopathy patients, a high-resolution technique to delineate those regions that are more likely to associate with sudden death will be critical. Hence, T1 mapping may provide a more reproducible and accurate method to delineate the PIR extent and variability, and as a result, the clinical risks imposed by the PIR.

T1 Mapping Sequences for Ischemic Cardiomyopathy

Several T1 mapping methods exist that all stem from an Inversion recovery (IR) and Look-Locker (LL) origin, but which have been improved with each iteration to achieve more rapid and reliable T1 maps. Based on these principles, modified Look-Locker methods (original and modified) and several saturation recovery methods have been developed (Fig. 6.2).

SMART1Map

The SMART1Map is an investigational pulse sequence that uses a single-point, saturation-recovery FIESTA acquisition to measure the T1 of myocardium. The pulse sequence also provides the ability to measure the duration of

each heartbeat in real time. In this sequence, each RR interval receives a saturation pulse with the acquisition of longer delay times in the recovery curve performed across multiple heart beats. This eliminates T1* correction and is less sensitive to other imaging parameters [10]. Saturation recovery times (TS) can be divided into two groups: (1) TS < T_{RR} and (2) TS > T_{RR}. Group 1 can be considered fixed saturation times because they are independent of heart rate variation during the scan (Fig. 6.3). The fixed TSs are determined by three factors: the prep time, trigger delay and the number of fixed TSs. The fixed saturation times are spaced evenly between prep time and trigger delay. The saturation recovery times in group 2 are heart-rate dependent. These are the heart-rate-dependent saturation times (TS > T_{RR}) and they use the trigger delay as a reference point [11].

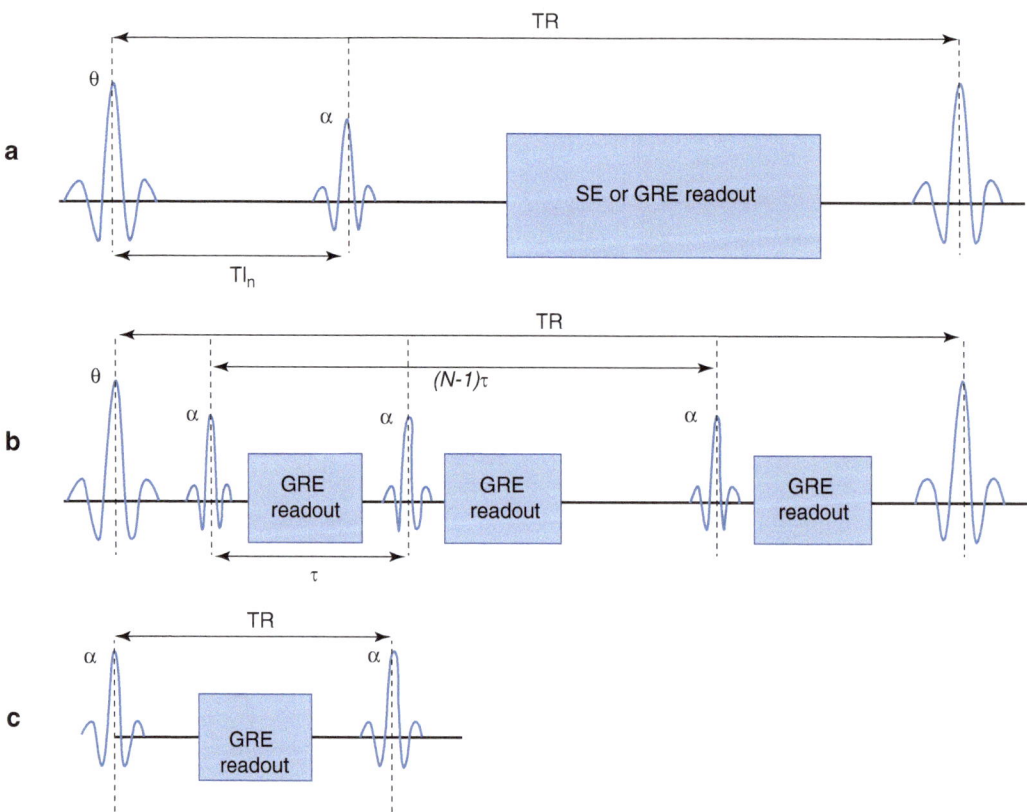

Fig. 6.2 Pulse sequences of common T1 mapping MRI strategies: (**a**) inversion recovery, (**b**) Look-Locker, (**c**) variable flip angle T1 mapping. Reprinted from [9]

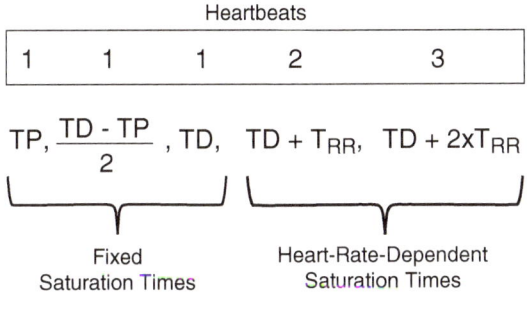

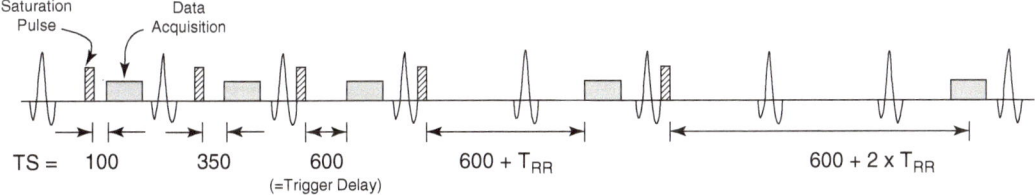

Fig. 6.3 Smart T1 mapping sequence as described by GE, Inc.

Combination of Intrinsic T1 Versus Contrast Agent-Enhanced T1 Mapping

Native

T1 mapping is an effective tool to characterize the histological changes in the myocardial tissues. Pathological changes, including fibrosis, necrosis and edema increase pre-contrast (native) T1 value of the myocardium. It contains both myocytes and connective tissue information. Native T1 mapping can be performed in patients with renal dysfunction. In ischemic cardiomyopathy, the value of native T1 mapping has not been clearly established, and typically it is combined with a post-contrast gadolinium enhanced T1, where it can be used to generate an ECV measurement.

Gadolinium (Gd)

The post-gadolinium T1 value of normal myocardium acquired between 10 and 15 min after infusion is significantly shorter than the pre-contrast T1 of normal myocardium [12]. Post-contrast T1 values of scarred or infarcted myocardium is significantly shorter than those of normal myocardium due to the retention of gadolinium in this fibrotic tissue, significantly higher ECV percentage, and lower flow state [13]. However, the existence of various factors that could affect post-contrast T1, such as the tissue status, hematocrit (Hct), the time delay after administration, and T1 mapping acquisition sequences, makes it difficult to assess myocardial fibrosis by itself [14]. To account for these variables, the ECV of the myocardium is calculated by measuring Hct and T1 for the blood pool: $ECV = (1 - Hct) \times (R1_{post} - R1_{pre})_{myo}/(R1_{post} - R1_{pre})_{blood}$, where R1 equals 1/T1 [15]. After bolus injection of gadolinium based agent, imaging is performed after at least 15 min from the injection, which generates equivalent results with the equilibrium contrast infusion [16]. ECV value is independent of field strength and may have more relevance in clinical practice [7, 17]. Expansion of the ECV fraction in the infarct injury region causes a greater change in the MRI relaxation (R1) value after the administration of the gadolinium-based extracellular contrast agent when compared to the remote myocardium [7, 18]. The extent of ECV changes could predict LV function and cardiovascular events following myocardial infarction

[19, 20]. The high risk DM patients showed a higher ECV value compared to the low risk patients [21].

Manganese (Mn)

In contrast to the native T1 and ECV mapping, quantification of manganese uptake into the cardiomyocytes through the voltage-gated calcium channels can produce direct representation of myocardial viability. Because of this property, Mn imaging generates a more accurate quantification of myocardial viability, which may predict future LV remodeling and arrhythmogenecity more sensitively in comparison to the Gd-based evaluation of cardiac fibrosis and extracellular volume (ECV) fraction. Delayed Gd-enhancement (DEMRI) is known to underestimate cardiac viability [22, 23]. In contrast, manganese-enhanced MRI (MEMRI) differentiates the non-viable infarct from viable myocardium and delineates the injured cardiomyocytes in the peri-infarct region. Our previous studies using dual contrast agents of gadolinium and manganese successfully identified the border zone around the infarct core, which contained injured but still viable myocardium (Fig. 6.4) [8, 24].

The significant changes in R1 value pre- and post MEMRI characterized the PIR more accurately by quantifying the myocardial viability. EVP 1001-1 (Eagle Vision Pharmaceutical, Corp, PA) is a cardiac-specific intracellular contrast agent that contains manganese and calcium with high safety profiles [25]. A short plasma half-life up to 1.5 min, rapid myocardial uptake, long retention time in the myocardium over 1 h, and no redistribution eliminates extracellular distribution. Reliable quantification of myocardium-specific manganese uptake is possible with minimal artifact from the timing of image acquisition [25, 26]. These features enable accurate quantification of myocardial viability of the infarct core and peri-infarct region through excellent spatial and temporal resolution.

Although manganese uptake by the myocardial tissue indicate the extent of viable cardiomyocytes, various factors could affect the uptake. Impaired calcium handling in heart failure could decrease manganese uptake. Stunned myocardium that is viable but dysfunctional shows decreased uptake of manganese and reduce delta R1 post MEMRI [27]. Higher heart rate and increased plasma level of neurohumoral factors up-regulate the uptake of manganese by cardiomyocytes (Fig. 6.5) [26].

Summary and Future Directions

As techniques continue to be refined for T1 mapping of the ischemic cardiomyopathy, the correlation of T1 map findings with clinical outcomes must follow. Our current tools to identify, quantify, and correlate PIR characteristics with arrhythmia, functional recovery, and overall prognosis are still developing, but early data suggest that there is a wealth of clinically valuable information within the PIR. The use of alternative contrast agents, specifically MEMRI, produces unique viability information about the PIR and may help define the clinical management of ischemic cardiomyopathy patients.

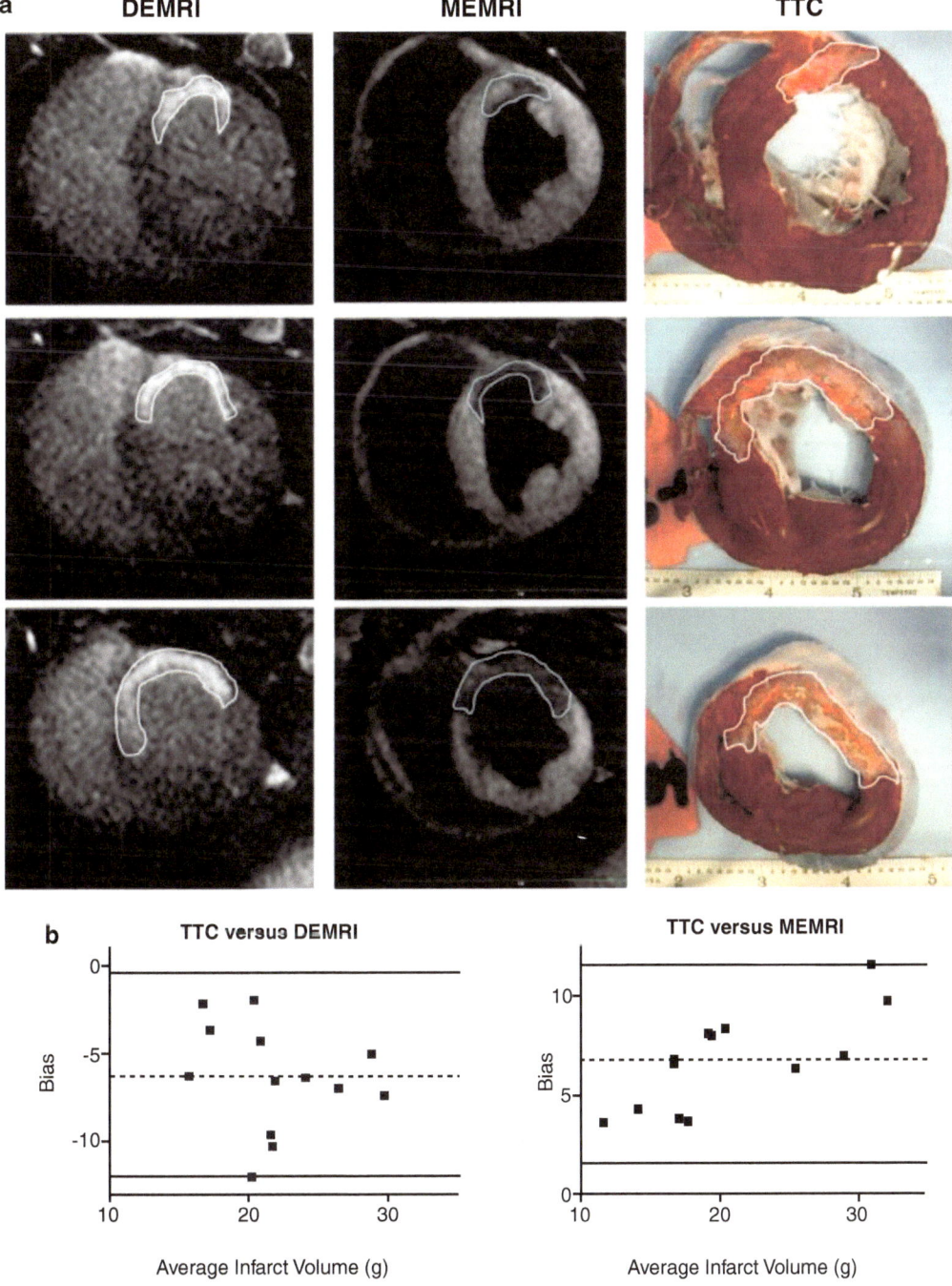

Fig. 6.4 Overlapping DEMRI and MEMRI signals denote viable border zone tissue and overestimated of infarct size with DEMRI. Reprinted from Dash et al. JACC CV Imaging 2011

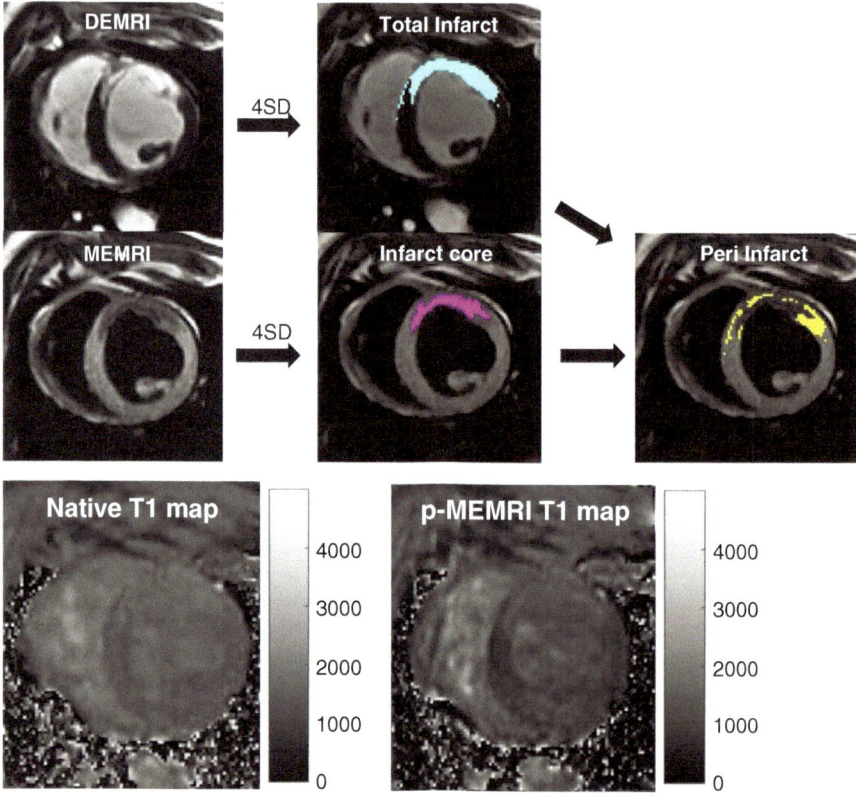

Fig. 6.5 PIR delineation & T1 mapping using gadolinium (DEMRI) versus manganese (MEMRI). Top images show sample short-axis DEMRI and MEMRI images of an anterior infarct with the typical bright T1 signal from DEMRI images and a corresponding signal void anteriorly in the MEMRI image of that slice. Using a semiautomatic tracing analysis of each image, the calculated infarct regions are noted and MEMRI void (true infarct) is subtracted from DEMRI total injury region to determine the peri-infarct region (PIR). Precontrast T1 Infarct core 1634.7 ± 88.4 ms, PIR 1530.5 ± 75.2 ms, Remote 1406.4 ± 37.9 ms (IC vs. PIR; p = 0.001, PIR vs. RR; p < 0.0001). Post MEMRI T1 Infarct core 1262.6 ± 126.8 ms, PIR 1136.3 ± 99.6 ms, Remote 956.7 ± 138.1 ms (IC vs. PIR; p = 0.005, PIR vs. RR; p = 0.0001). Delta R1 Infarct core 0.18 ± 0.09 s⁻¹, PIR 0.23 ± 0.08 s⁻¹, Remote 0.35 ± 0.19 s⁻¹ (IC vs. PIR; p = 0.04, PIR vs. RR = 0.01). Tada et al.

References

1. Bunch TJ, Hohnloser SH, Gersh BJ. Mechanisms of sudden cardiac death in myocardial infarction survivors: insights from the randomized trials of implantable cardioverter-defibrillators. Circulation. 2007;115(18):2451–7.
2. Solomon SD, Zelenkofske S, McMurray JJ, Finn PV, Velazquez E, Ertl G, Harsanyi A, Rouleau JL, Maggioni A, Kober L, White H, Van de Werf F, Pieper K, Califf RM, Pfeffer MA, Investigators V i AMITV. Sudden death in patients with myocardial infarction and left ventricular dysfunction, heart failure, or both. N Engl J Med. 2005;352(25):2581–8.
3. Schuleri KH, Centola M, George RT, Amado LC, Evers KS, Kitagawa K, Vavere AL, Evers R, Hare JM, Cox C, McVeigh ER, Lima JA, Lardo AC. Characterization of peri-infarct zone heterogeneity by contrast-enhanced multidetector computed tomographya comparison with magnetic resonance imaging. J Am Coll Cardiol. 2009;53(18):1699–707.
4. Heidary S, Patel H, Chung J, Yokota H, Gupta SN, Bennett MV, Katikireddy C, Nguyen P, Pauly JM, Terashima M, McConnell MV, Yang PC. Quantitative tissue characterization of infarct core and border zone in patients with ischemic cardiomyopathy by magnetic resonance is associated with future cardiovascular events. J Am Coll Cardiol. 2010;55(24):2762–8.
5. Kim RJ, Wu E, Rafael A, Chen EL, Parker MA, Simonetti O, Klocke FJ, Bonow RO, Judd RM. The use of contrast-enhanced magnetic resonance imaging to identify reversible myocardial dysfunction. N Engl J Med. 2000;343(20):1445–53.

6. Yokota H, Heidary S, Katikireddy CK, Nguyen P, Pauly JM, McConnell MV, Yang PC. Quantitative characterization of myocardial infarction by cardiovascular magnetic resonance predicts future cardiovascular events in patients with ischemic cardiomyopathy. J Cardiovasc Magn Reson. 2008;10:17.

7. Ugander M, Oki AJ, Hsu LY, Kellman P, Greiser A, Aletras AH, Sibley CT, Chen MY, Bandettini WP, Arai AE. Extracellular volume imaging by magnetic resonance imaging provides insights into overt and sub-clinical myocardial pathology. Eur Heart J. 2012;33(10):1268–78.

8. Dash R, Chung J, Ikeno F, Hahn-Windgassen A, Matsuura Y, Bennett MV, Lyons JK, Teramoto T, Robbins RC, McConnell MV, Yeung AC, Brinton TJ, Harnish PP, Yang PC. Dual manganese-enhanced and delayed gadolinium-enhanced MRI detects myocardial border zone injury in a pig ischemia-reperfusion model. Circ Cardiovasc Imaging. 2011;4(5):574–82.

9. Stikov N, Tardif C, Barral J, Levesque I, Pike B. T1 mapping: methods & challenges. 2011 ISMRM annual meeting, Montreal, Canada. 2011.

10. Moon JC, Messroghli DR, Kellman P, Piechnik SK, Robson MD, Ugander M, Gatehouse PD, Arai AE, Friedrich MG, Neubauer S, Schulz-Menger J, Schelbert EB, Imaging S f CMR, Cardiology CMRWG o t ES o. Myocardial T1 mapping and extracellular volume quantification: a Society for Cardiovascular Magnetic Resonance (SCMR) and CMR Working Group of the European Society of Cardiology consensus statement. J Cardiovasc Magn Reson. 2013;15:92.

11. Dandekar VK, Bauml MA, Ertel AW, Dickens C, Gonzalez RC, Farzaneh-Far A. Assessment of global myocardial perfusion reserve using cardiovascular magnetic resonance of coronary sinus flow at 3 Tesla. J Cardiovasc Magn Reson. 2014;16.24.

12. Messroghli DR, Plein S, Higgins DM, Walters K, Jones TR, Ridgway JP, Sivananthan MU. Human myocardium: single-breath-hold MR T1 mapping with high spatial resolution—reproducibility study. Radiology. 2006;238(3):1004–12.

13. Messroghli DR, Walters K, Plein S, Sparrow P, Friedrich MG, Ridgway JP, Sivananthan MU. Myocardial T1 mapping: application to patients with acute and chronic myocardial infarction. Magn Reson Med. 2007;58(1):34–40.

14. Mewton N, Liu CY, Croisille P, Bluemke D, Lima JA. Assessment of myocardial fibrosis with cardiovascular magnetic resonance. J Am Coll Cardiol. 2011;57(8):891–903.

15. Flett AS, Hayward MP, Ashworth MT, Hansen MS, Taylor AM, Elliott PM, McGregor C, Moon JC. Equilibrium contrast cardiovascular magnetic resonance for the measurement of diffuse myocardial fibrosis: preliminary validation in humans. Circulation. 2010;122(2):138–44.

16. Schelbert EB, Testa SM, Meier CG, Ceyrolles WJ, Levenson JE, Blair AJ, Kellman P, Jones BL, Ludwig DR, Schwartzman D, Shroff SG, Wong TC. Myocardial extravascular extracellular volume fraction measurement by gadolinium cardiovascular magnetic resonance in humans: slow infusion versus bolus. J Cardiovasc Magn Reson. 2011;13:16.

17. Kellman P, Wilson JR, Xue H, Ugander M, Arai AE. Extracellular volume fraction mapping in the myocardium, part 1: evaluation of an automated method. J Cardiovasc Magn Reson. 2012;14:63.

18. Wendland MF. Applications of manganese-enhanced magnetic resonance imaging (MEMRI) to imaging of the heart. NMR Biomed. 2004;17(8):581–94.

19. Kidambi A, Motwani M, Uddin A, Ripley DP, McDiarmid AK, Swoboda PP, Broadbent DA, Musa TA, Erhayiem B, Leader J, Croisille P, Clarysse P, Greenwood JP, Plein S. Myocardial extracellular volume estimation by CMR predicts functional recovery following acute MI. JACC Cardiovasc Imaging. 2017;10(9):989–99.

20. Messroghli DR, Moon JC, Ferreira VM, Grosse-Wortmann L, He T, Kellman P, Mascherbauer J, Nezafat R, Salerno M, Schelbert EB, Taylor AJ, Thompson R, Ugander M, van Heeswijk RB, Friedrich MG. Clinical recommendations for cardiovascular magnetic resonance mapping of T1, T2, T2* and extracellular volume: a consensus statement by the Society for Cardiovascular Magnetic Resonance (SCMR) endorsed by the European Association for Cardiovascular Imaging (EACVI). J Cardiovasc Magn Reson. 2017;19(1):75.

21. Gai N, Turkbey EB, Nazarian S, van der Geest RJ, Liu CY, Lima JA, Bluemke DA. T1 mapping of the gadolinium-enhanced myocardium: adjustment for factors affecting interpatient comparison. Magn Reson Med. 2011;65(5):1407–15.

22. Saeed M, Bremerich J, Wendland MF, Wyttenbach R, Weinmann HJ, Higgins CB. Reperfused myocardial infarction as seen with use of necrosis-specific versus standard extracellular MR contrast media in rats. Radiology. 1999;213(1):247–57.

23. Saeed M, Lund G, Wendland MF, Bremerich J, Weinmann H, Higgins CB. Magnetic resonance characterization of the peri-infarction zone of reperfused myocardial infarction with necrosis-specific and extracellular nonspecific contrast media. Circulation. 2001;103(6):871–6.

24. Dash R, Kim PJ, Matsuura Y, Ikeno F, Metzler S, Huang NF, Lyons JK, Nguyen PK, Ge X, Foo CW, McConnell MV, Wu JC, Yeung AC, Harnish P, Yang PC. Manganese-enhanced magnetic resonance imaging enables in vivo confirmation of peri-infarct restoration following stem cell therapy in a porcine ischemia-reperfusion model. J Am Heart Assoc. 2015;4(7).

25. Storey P, Danias PG, Post M, Li W, Seoane PR, Harnish PP, Edelman RR, Prasad PV. Preliminary evaluation of EVP 1001-1: a new cardiac-specific magnetic resonance contrast agent with kinetics suitable for steady-state imaging of the ischemic heart. Investig Radiol. 2003;38(10):642–52.

26. Eriksson R, Johansson L, Bjerner T, Ahlström H. Dobutamine-induced stress affects intracellular uptake of manganese: a quantitative magnetic resonance imaging study in pigs. J Magn Reson Imaging. 2005;21(4):360–4.

27. Krombach GA, Saeed M, Higgins CB, Novikov V, Wendland MF. Contrast-enhanced MR delineation of stunned myocardium with administration of MnCl(2) in rats. Radiology. 2004;230(1):183–90.

T1 Mapping in Stem Cell Therapy

7

Yoko Kato, Mohammad R. Ostovaneh,
Bharath Ambale-Venkatesh, and Joao Lima

Cardiac Disease and Stem Cell Therapy (Overview of the Previous Stem Cell Studies)

Cell therapy is a novel technique to recover myocardial function by reverse remodeling. It is also referred to as "Cellular cardiomyoplasty" [1]. In general, cell therapy deploys stem cells to the damaged myocardium by cell delivery methods of direct myocardial injection (during surgery), transcatheter endomyocardial injection (TESI) [2, 3], or intracoronary injection (IC).

Stem cell therapy has been used to target a broad range of cardiomyopathies. These include ischemic heart disease (IHD) like acute myocardial infarction (AMI) [4–7], or chronic ischemic heart disease (IHD) [8, 9], or non-ischemic cardiomyopathies (NICMs) like dilated cardiomy-

opathy [10–13], or drug-induced cardiomyopathy (Table 7.1).

Several types of cells have been developed and used in clinical trials. Cells with limited regenerative potential like bone marrow cells (BMCs) and mesenchymal stem cells [14] were used in the early years of stem cell study. These heterogeneous cell populations have been called "first-generation" stem cells, in contrast to contemporary "second-generation" counterparts with high regenerative potential [15]. The latter consist of more purified cell populations with a presumed greater potential for cardiac repair and are often derived from non-bone marrow sources, or subjected to genetic and pharmacological "priming" in vitro to enhance their engraftment, survival, plasticity, and paracrine activity. In the second generation, cardiosphere derived cells (CDCs) [7], c-kit positive cells [8], embryonic stem cells and induced pluripotent stem cells are reported [15]. The safety of stem cell therapies have now been established by many previous studies.

Autologous cells were deployed in early studies, but the efficacy of allogeneic compared to autologous cells has been also studied in several recent reports. The extraction and production of autologous cells are more difficult than allogenic cells. So far, allogeneic cells have shown a comparable safety profile. The effect on myocardial function recovery, measured using ejection fraction or wall motion, using allogeneic as compared

Y. Kato · M. R. Ostovaneh
Department of Cardiology, Johns Hopkins University School of Medicine, Baltimore, MD, USA
e-mail: ykato8@jhmi.edu; mostova1@jhmi.edu

B. Ambale-Venkatesh (✉)
Department of Radiology, Johns Hopkins University School of Medicine, Baltimore, MD, USA
e-mail: bambale1@jhu.edu

J. Lima
Department of Cardiology, Johns Hopkins University School of Medicine, Baltimore, MD, USA

Department of Radiology, Johns Hopkins University School of Medicine, Baltimore, MD, USA
e-mail: jlima@jhmi.edu

© Springer International Publishing AG, part of Springer Nature 2018
P. C. Yang (ed.), *T1-Mapping in Myocardial Disease*, https://doi.org/10.1007/978-3-319-91110-6_7

Table 7.1 Previous studies on stem cell therapy

Study	First author	year	Disease	Treatment	Injection method	Cell source and type	Autograft/allograft
BOOST [4]	Wollert	2004	STEMI	PCI + BMC IC	IC	BMC	Autograft
ASTAMI [5]	Lunde	2006	STEMI	PCI + BMC IC	IC	BMC	Autograft
HEBE [6]	Hirsch	2011	First STEMI	PCI + cells IC	IC	Mononuclear cells from BM or peripheral blood in patients	Autograft
CADUCEUS [7]	Malliaras	2014	AMI <4W, LVEF 25–45%	PCI + CDC IC	IC	CDCs	Autograft
SCIPIO [8],	Bolli	2011	ICM LVEF ≤40% planned CABG	CABG+ (4M post CABG) CSC IC	IC	c-kit-positive CSCs	Autograft
TAC-HFT [9]	Heldman	2014	ICM LVEF <50%	MSC/BMC	TESI	MSCs and BMCs	Autograft
TOPCARE-DCM [10]	Fischer-Rasokat	2009	DCM LVEF <40%, LVDd >60 mm	BMC IC	IC	BMC	Autograft
ABCD [11]	Seth	2010	DCM LVEF <40%	BMC IC	IC	BMC	Autograft
NOGA-DCM [12]	Vrtovec	2013	DCM	BMC	TESI vs. IC	BMC	Autograft
POSEIDON-DCM [13]	Hare	2017	DCM LVEF <40%, LVDd >5.9 cm (Male) or >5.6 cm (Female), or and LVEDV index >125 mL/m²	Allo-hMSC vs. auto-hMSC transendocardial injection at 10 LV sites	TESI	hMSCs	Autograft or allograft

N (intervention/control group)	Duration of f/u	Results	Main parameters	Echocardiography	SPECT	LVG	Cine MRI	LGE
30/30	6M	Positive	LVEF (LGE no effect)				1	1
50/50	6M	Negative	LVEF (SPECT), infarct size		1 (LVEF, infarct size)		1	1
BMCs/mononuclear peripheral blood cells/standard therapy (without placebo infusion) 69/65/65	4M	Negative	LVEF, dysfunctional LV segments, LV volume, mass, infarct size	1			1	1
17/8	12M	Positive and negative (scar size decreased, LVEF no difference)	LVEF, scar (MRI or CT)				1	1 (or CT)
16/7	12M	Positive	LVEF, infarct size (LGE) measured in treatment subgroup	1			1	1 (only for 7 stem cell patients)
MSC 22/11 BMC 22/10	12M	MSCs positive in circumferential strain. Negative in chamber volume and EF	Infarct size, strain, LVEF, chamber volume				1	1 (or CT)
33 (no control group)	3M	Positive	LVEF, wall motion	1			subgroup (9)	
41/40	36M	Positive	LVEF	1				
20 (TESI)/20 (IC)	6M	TESI vs. IC, TESI better in LVEF	LVEF	1				
19(allo)/18(auto)	12M	Comparison of Auto/Allo	LVEF, 6MWT, NYHA classification				1 (or CT)	

SPECT single-photon-emission computed tomography, *LVG* left ventriculography, *MRI* magnetic resonance imaging, *LGE* late gadolinium enhancement, *STEMI* ST elevation myocardial infarction, *PCI* percutaneous coronary intervention. *BMC* bone marrow cell, *IC* intracoronary, *CDC* cardiosphere-derived cell, *CABG* coronary aorta bypass graft, *ICM* ischemic cardiomyopathy, *MSC* mesenchymal stem cell, *TESI* transendocardial stem cell injection, *EF* ejection fraction, *CT* computed tomography, *DCM* diastolic cardiomyopathy, *LVDd* left ventricular diastolic dimension, *LVEDV* left ventricular end-diastolic volume, *6MWT* 6 minutes-walk test, *NYHA* New York Heart Association, *BM* bone marrow, *CSC* cardiac stem cells, *hMSC* human mesenchymal stem cell, *LV* left ventricular to autologous cells is an active area of research. So far, the superiority of autograft/allograft cells are inconsistent and there are several considerations [13, 16].

The goal of stem cell therapy is the functional recovery of the heart and prognostic improvement. For the functional assessment of endpoints, imaging modalities such as echocardiography, left ventriculography (LVG), single-photon-emission computed tomography (SPECT), computed tomography (CT), and cardiac magnetic resonance imaging (MRI) have been used. For the assessment of myocardial tissue characteristics, SPECT or cardiac MRI late gadolinium enhancement (LGE) have generally been used. Some previous studies have assessed the same patients with different modalities and compared the results. Cardiac MRI is generally accepted as the gold standard modality for assessment of changes in myocardial function and tissue characteristics because of the excellent reproducibility it affords as well as the improved spatial resolution that allows quantification and characterization at the millimeter-level. MRI also is completely non-invasive and performs imaging using non-ionizing radiation, and carries no known long-term risks to patients.

Ischemic (AMI/Chronic Ischemia)

Ischemic heart disease has been one of the important targets in stem cell therapy. The main endpoint studied in previous reports has been an increase in left ventricular ejection fraction (LVEF), but the results so far have been fairly inconsistent, with the effects limited. Preservation of the LVEF is generally one of the last functional indices that change throughout the disease process. One of the reasons might be that the endpoint of LVEF might not be specific to improvement in myocardial function with effects from other factors such as loading conditions and concomitant disease conditions. We may need to detect more subtle changes of myocardial function like diastolic function, strain, or torsion, especially when we think about the well-known

ischemic cascade [17], a complex biological process, which stem cell therapy must reverse.

Previous Studies on AMI: BOOST [4], ASTAMI [5], HEBE [6], CADUCEUS [7] (Table 7.1)

There have been several trials looking into the effect of various cell types in patients with a variety of cardiac diseases. A few of them have used MRI measured cardiac structure, function, and morphology as the endpoints. The BOne marrOw transfer to enhance ST-elevation infarct regeneration (the BOOST) trial [4] was a randomized trial conducted between years 2002–2003 that reported the potential beneficial effects of stem cells in the first 6 months after therapy. The primary endpoint was LVEF assessed on MRI. At 6 months, LVEF increased significantly in the cell (injected with bone marrow derived cells (BMCs)) group compared to the control group (6.7% vs. 0.7%, $p = 0.0026$). However, at 18 months, LVEF did now show a sustained improvement and overall, the mean LVEF change in 18 months did not show significant difference between the groups [18]. This study suggests the difficulty of setting a suitable follow-up period as well as relying on LVEF alone as a viable endpoint to understand the underlying pathophysiology.

ASTAMI (Autologous Stem cell Transplantation in Acute Myocardial Infarction) trial [5] was also a randomized controlled trial in which patients with acute myocardial infarction were injected BMC cell type or placebo 6 days after hospitalization. End points included changes in the LVEF and infarct size. They assessed LVEF with three modalities, including SPECT, echocardiography, and MRI, and the infarct size with SPECT and late gadolinium enhancement (LGE). At 6 months, all the patients showed LVEF increase of 7.6 ± 10.4%, but when LVEF change was compared between the treatment and control groups, there was no significant difference as assessed by any modalities. The treatment group did not differ significantly from control group in infarct size assessed on SPECT or LGE when compared with the baseline and the 6 months. Acute MI is a setting where dynamic changes happen to the structure and function of the heart, and therefore the choice of LVEF, in particular, could be fraught with difficulties in trying to separate natural changes immediately after MI from the cell therapy effects. Scar size measured by LGE is also seen to decrease in the immediate days and months following MI before stabilizing, yet LGE alone is non-specific for small changes in scar size that occurs with stem cell therapy, particularly in the peri-infarct region.

HEBE trial [6] was a randomized trial that also reported negative results. Their target disease was large first AMI treated with PCI. They randomly assigned the patients to mononuclear BMCs (n = 69), mononuclear peripheral blood cells (n = 66), or standard therapy (without placebo infusion) (n = 65). In 4 months, they found that intracoronary infusion of cell therapy did not improve regional or global systolic myocardial function. They have assessed the infarct size using LGE, but there was no significant difference in the amount of infarct size reduction among the groups. This study suggests the importance of follow up period to assess the efficacy of stem cell therapy. As they discussed in the paper, follow-up MRI at 4 months was too early to detect the changes in LV function and remodeling and long term consequences of treatment may have been missed. There are two very important considerations relevant to the design of the cell therapy trials: timeline for recovery from hibernation, and also to detect the reverse-remodeling from cell therapy intervention. Moreover, given that the effect size in cell therapy trials is expected to be small, accurate and reproducible methods are to be considered for endpoint assessment.

CADUCEUS (CArdiosphere-Derived aUtologous stem CElls to reverse ventricUlar dySfunction) trial [7] was a prospective, randomized, controlled trial that showed improvement in scar size by LGE, but not in LVEF. The target disease was AMI within 4 weeks with successful PCI and LVEF of 25–45%. They deployed autologous cardiosphere-derived cells (CDCs) harvested from the biopsy sample of endomyocardium. At 1 year, CDC-treated patients had smaller scar size on LGE compared with control patients, while no differences in the change of LVEF were observed between CDC-treated patients (5.4 ± 10.6%) and control patients (5.8 ± 3.3%, p = 0.636 between groups). Interestingly, at the regional level, myocardial segments treated with CDCs showed improved segmental wall thickening and circumferential strain although this did not translate to improvement in LVEF. The improvement in regional function was correlated with reduction in scar size by LGE. The significant difference seen in LGE but not in LVEF, together with the improvement in regional function, suggests that the LVEF may not be the best index to detect the effect size in cell therapy trials.

One limitation of these studies is rather short follow-up period and the lack of data on long-term prognosis of patients treated with stem cells. For an example, it is not well understood whether the patients with unchanged LVEF, improved regional function and reduced scar and fibrosis have better long-term prognosis when compared to their counterparts with similar LVEF but worse regional function and greater scar burden. Currently there is a large scale ongoing study on efficacy of BMCs on AMI, "the phase III BAMI trial" with the initial sample size of 3000 participants (reduced to 400), which is expected to shed light into many of unanswered questions in the field. This trial is aiming for completion by May 2018 [19].

Previous Studies on Chronic Ischemia: SCIPIO [8], **TAC-HFT** [9] (Table 7.1)

SCIPIO (Stem Cell Infusion in Patients with Ischemic cardiomyopathy) [8] was a small phase 1 study that showed positive results in LVEF recovery. Patients with post-infarction LV dysfunction (ejection fraction [EF] ≤40%) before coronary artery bypass grafting were included. Cardiac stem cells (CSCs) expressing the surface receptor tyrosine kinase c-kit was utilized. Treatment group patients received IC injection of c-kit positive (surface tyrosine kinase receptor) cardiac stem cells (CaSC) 4 months after CABG. Four months after CaSCs infusion, LVEF increased from 30.3% (SE 1.9) to 38.5% (2.8, p = 0.001) while in control patients LVEF did not change (30.1% (2.4) to 30.2% (2.5)). They also reported decreased infarct size on LGE in small subgroup (N = 7) of treated patients although none of the control group participants underwent LGE and placebo effect could not be ruled out. The advantage of the SCIPIO trial was allowing 4 months after revascularization to eliminate the effect of recovery from hibernation even though the follow-up time after cell therapy was relatively short for the assessment of persistence of treatment effect.

TAC-HFT [9] was a study that showed reduction in infarct size and improvement in circumferential strain but failed to demonstrate any improvement in LVEF or LV size. This trial was a phase 1 and 2 randomized, blinded, placebo-controlled study that included 65 patients with ischemic cardiomyopathy and LVEF less than 50%. The study compared MSCs (n = 19) with placebo (n = 11) and BMCs (n = 19) with placebo (n = 10) and all patients were followed up for 1 year. Infarct size was significantly reduced with MSCs (−18.9%; 95% CI, −30.4 to −7.4; within-group, P = 0.004) but not with BMCs compared to placebo. Also, regional myocardial function indexed as peak circumferential strain at the site of injection improved with MSCs (−4.9; 95% CI, −13.3 to 3.5; within-group repeated measures, P = 0.03) but not with BMCs. Similar to most of other studies, no change in LVEF or LV size was observed in this study.

Non-ischemic (DCM/Other Non-ischemic Pathology): TOPCARE-DCM [10], ABCD [11], NOGA-DCM [12], POSEIDON-DCM [13] (Table 7.1)

Cell therapy trials in non-ischemic cardiomyopathies are scarce in the literature and the most of those few studies are focused on dilated cardiomyopathy (DCM). There is also an ongoing study to assess the efficacy of cell therapy in Duchenne muscular dystrophy (HOPE trial, NCT02485938) with expected study completion by late 2017. In contrast to ischemic cardiomyopathy, the etiology of injury in non-ischemic cardiomyopathy is not ischemia driven. Mechanism of action for cell therapy might, therefore, differ from ischemic cardiomyopathy.

TOPCARE-DCM (Transplantation of Progenitor Cells and Recovery of Left Ventricular Function in Patients with non-ischemic Dilated Cardiomyopathy) [10] was a pilot study that tested the efficacy of IC injection of BMCs in DCM patients with reduced LVEF <40% and dilated LV (LVDd >60 mm). The study demonstrated improved LVEF at 3-months follow-up after cell injection. However, there was no placebo group in this trial.

ABCD [11] was another open-label, randomized study that showed promising results for patients with DCM. Eighty one patients with DCM were enrolled in the study and were randomized to either IC injection of BMCs (n = 41) and control (n = 40). Three years of follow-up period demonstrated that the LVEF significantly improved in the treated patients by 5.9% but there was no change in LVEF in the control arm. The power of this study to demonstrated that the improved LVEF might be most likely attributed to unchanged end-diastolic volume, which attenuates the load dependence of LVEF in this study.

NOGA-DCM [12] was an open-label blinded study that compared stem cell through TESI or IC routes in DCM patients. Peripheral blood stem cells that express CD34+ and are labeled with 99m Tc-hexamethylpropyleneamine oxime were administered. Eighteen hours after cell administration, the retention rate was higher in TESI group (19.2 ± 4.8% vs. 4.4 ± 1.2%, P < 0.01). At 6 months, LVEF on echocardiography improved more in the TESI group (+8.1 ± 4.3%) compared to IC group (+4.2 ± 2.3%, P = 0.03). The study concluded that in patients with non-ischemic DCM, CD34+ cell transplantation through TESI route is associated with higher cell retention rate and greater improvement in ventricular function, NT-proBNP levels, and exercise capacity compared with the IC route.

POSEIDON-DCM [13] was a randomized trial, comparing the safety and efficacy of autologous (auto) versus allogeneic (allo) human bone marrow-derived mesenchymal stem cells (hMSCs) in non-ischemic DCM. The study demonstrated that the allogeneic hMSCs are superior to autologous hMSCs to improve LVEF, 6-minutes walk test and Minnesota Living with Heart Failure Questionnaire (MLHFQ). This study was noted for particular importance in using the allogenic stem cells in DCM, given the less complex administration of the allogeneic versus autologous cells.

Endpoint Determination in Stem Cell Therapy

The effect of stem cell therapy is an active area of research (Table 7.1). Some of the results from the prior studies while beneficial in many cases were also not consistent across all studies. There may be several reasons for this discrepancy, including cell characteristics, delivery methods, and follow-up periods. Therefore, we will discuss the role of choosing optimal endpoints particularly as it relates to imaging.

Left Ventricular Ejection Fraction

LVEF has been the end-point of choice in prior stem cell therapy trials. LVEF is easy to measure, can be obtained using a number of imaging modalities, and easily analyzed and interpreted. It has been the gold-standard clinical end-point for over 60 years. For these reasons, it is most often chosen as the primary analysis of interest in cardiomyopathy trials.

Madonna et al. have discussed several limitations of cell-based therapy. They pointed out two limitations related to image analysis: (1) the use of LVEF for assessing the effects of cell therapy and (2) incorrect target population with modest baseline LVEF reduction ~50% who generally hold a favorable outcome [15, 20].

Henry et al. have also discussed the inconsistency of the results of stem cell therapy [21]. One of the discussion points was the difficulty in identifying high-risk patients. LVEF alone (especially early LVEF) is inadequate because of myocardial stunning. Another point was the difficulty of differentiating the cell-based efficacy from that

derived from successful reperfusion treatment due to the hibernating myocardium after STEMI. Also, the study pointed out the limitation of MRI, such as limitation of LGE to differentiate true infarction scar from myocardial edema, or the significant drop-out rate derived from claustrophobia or device (defibrillators and pacemakers) related limitation to undergo MRI. They referred the significant drop-out rate from MRI of 25% in SWISS-AMI trial [22].

The use of LVEF may be a major limitation in stem cell studies. The studies indicate the importance to recognize that the LVEF may not be an ideal indicator of myocardial improvement and identification of the target population, using LVEF alone, might not be the best strategy. This discrepancy is evidenced by prior studies showing a poor correlation between NYHA functional class and the patient's LVEF.

LVEF has been the main parameter to describe cardiac function in previous studies (Table 7.1). While most previous trials have centered around the use of LVEF as the endpoint, LVEF may not be sensitive enough to assess subtle functional changes derived from stem cell therapy. According to the ischemic cascade [17], an increase in LVEF is likely a drastic change in cardiac function, compared to other more subtle functional changes such as diastolic function or myocardial strain. Moreover, several studies have noted how LVEF may not be the best prognosticator of cardiac morbidity and mortality [23, 24]. LVEF depends on a variety of factors including loading conditions, ventricular-arterial coupling, valve function, etc. in addition to myocardial function. As a result, subtle changes to myocardial health may not be correctly reflected in the quantified LVEF. A more obvious case of this is heart failure with preserved ejection fraction (HFpEF) where maintaining a normal or mildly reduced ejection fraction does not confer reduced risk. Indeed, patients with HFpEF have comparable mortality risk to those with heart failure with reduced ejection fraction (HFrEF). It is in this setting that a more compelling cardiac endpoint, which reflects the underlying myocardial tissue morphology would be beneficial, not only as a more accurate representation of the underlying myocardial biology but also independent of extraneous factors.

There are several measures such as myocardial strain and diastolic function, both measured from echocardiography and MRI, that are likely to be more sensitive and specific measures than LVEF and track better with myocardial tissue characteristics. These measures, however, are also not completely free of extraneous factors such as the loading conditions.

Previous studies by Iles et al. reported that post-contrast myocardial T1 time progressively shortened with worsening grades of diastolic function as assessed by echocardiography in patients with heart failure [25]. Echocardiography has its limitations of moderate reproducibility and inter-observer variability while cardiac MRI has better accuracy and reproducibility [26]. Combining diastolic function assessment with T1 mapping may give us more detailed information on cardiac function. Based on these observations, cardiac MRI is accepted as the most preferred modality in stem cell therapy.

Late Gadolinium Enhancement

LGE has been a well-established gold standard to assess focal myocardial fibrosis associated with damaged or scarred myocardium. Significant prognostic capability has been demonstrated in many previous studies in different patient populations such as in ischemic patients [25, 27, 28] and in non-ischemic diseases such as DCM [29, 30], HCM [31], and cardiac sarcoidosis [32]. Assessment of fibrosis using LGE adds several advantages as it relates to the efficacy of stem cell therapy and to the prognostic capability. Several stem cell therapies purport to either repair damaged myocardium by enhancing reparative mechanisms by improved paracrine activity or by replacing or reprogramming the cells in the damaged myocardium with viable cardiomyocytes. The use of LGE allows us to study not only the effect of cell therapies but also the mechanisms associated detailed myocardial T1-maps with areas of myocardial scarring clearly delineated. This also enables us to answer questions related

to identifying the optimal site and method of cell delivery. This is key in a fast-evolving field such as cell therapy where there are several different cell types and cell delivery methods. In addition, LGE allows a careful selection of the appropriate patient population to clinical trials as the subjects can now be enrolled based on the quantitative measurement of myocardial damage. Therefore, the assessment of myocardial fibrosis by LGE confers significant advances and complements LVEF measurement.

However, LGE has several limitations. It is difficult to differentiate scar from extracellular edema [33] so that in patients who sustain ischemic injury, LGE assessment may not uniquely refer to damaged tissue alone. Another weakness lies in the detection of diffuse fibrosis such as that observed in DCM [34], anthracycline-induced cardiotoxicity [35], or even in ischemic diseases in areas of peri-infarct region [25, 36]. For example, in DCM patients, about a third of the patients show characteristic mid-wall enhancement while the rest of them show negative LGE [30]. The effects of cardiotoxic drugs such as anthracycline-induced cardiomyopathy are often reported to have negative LGE due to the inability to detect early myocardial damage, which precedes LVEF reduction [35].

In patients with prior MI, the peri-infarct region surrounding the core myocardial scar consists of normal and fibrotic tissues, which leads to potential multiple re-entry circuits and arrhythmia and ventricular remodeling. The LGE of 'gray zone' in the peri-infarct region is observed as the area with lower signal intensity around the infarcted necrotic area. Previous studies by Yan et al. suggested that the extent of this gray zone provides additional prognostic information for cardiovascular mortality when compared to LVEF or LV systolic volume [25]. However, precise 'gray zone' detection techniques are not straightforward.

LGE also has several technical limitations. The measurement of fibrosis, using LGE, depends on several factors related to the contrast agent, administered dose, and timing of image acquisition. LGE imaging is also ineffective in detecting diffuse interstitial fibrosis seen in many disease processes, as well as in assessment of the gray zone. Additionally, accurate LGE quantification in the context of diffuse or patchy fibrosis can be very difficult. In order to address these limitations, which are critical in assessing stem cell therapy, T1 mapping provides critical information.

Cardiac Disease Assessment with T1 Mapping

Implication of Myocardial Fibrosis

Fibrosis can be roughly classified into three categories—Reactive fibrosis, infiltrative interstitial fibrosis, and replacement scar fibrosis. Reactive interstitial fibrosis is generally observed in hypertension, valvular disease, diabetes, genetic abnormality, or aging. It has a progressive onset and follows the increase in collagen synthesis by myofibroblasts under the influence of different stimuli. It is seen as an intermediate marker of disease severity and, generally, precedes irreversible replacement fibrosis.

Infiltrative interstitial fibrosis is seen in cases where deposits such as amyloidosis or glycosphingolipids (Anderson-Fabry disease) are in the cardiac interstitium. Replacement scar fibrosis replaces the myocytes after cell damage or necrosis by plexiform fibrosis, mainly type I collagen. This type of fibrosis can have a localized distribution such as acute/chronic ischemia, infarction, myocarditis, HCM, or cardiac sarcoidosis. It can also have a diffuse distribution like toxic cardiomyopathies or inflammatory diseases according to the underlying etiology. Infiltrative interstitial fibrosis and infiltrative fibrosis ultimately lead to replacement fibrosis in the later stages of disease where cellular damage and cardiomyocyte necrosis/apoptosis appear [36, 37].

T1 mapping has the potential to be clinically diagnostic modality to assess the diffuse fibrosis that LGE cannot reliably detect. There are four parameters generally used in the T1 mapping assessment: native T1, post-contrast T1, partition coefficient, and extracellular volume (ECV).

Native T1 refers to the T1 time in the absence of an exogenous contrast agent, which is the time constant representing the recovery of longitudinal magnetization (spin–lattice relaxation). It measures the T1 values from the composite of extracellular and intracellular compartments. Post-contrast T1 mapping refers to the T1 time in the presence of an exogenous contrast agent. Measuring the ratio of T1 changes pre and post contrast administration in the myocardium and blood provides the partition coefficient. When corrected by hematocrit the myocardial ECV is derived [38]. Combining the native T1 and ECV measurements, T1 mapping may act as a useful guide to differentiate the complex cardiomyopathic diseases [36, 39, 40].

T1 Mapping

Here, we look at a few different studies that have used T1 mapping for disease diagnosis and prognostication. T1 mapping in Multi-Ethnic Study of Atherosclerosis (MESA) study subjects was assessed and reported in age-related fibrosis [41], sex-associated differences in community without cardiovascular event history [42], ECG changes and myocardial fibrosis [43], and patients with cardiovascular disease risk factors [44]. Other studies have also studied the use of T1 mapping in STEMI [45, 46], DCM [34, 47], anthracycline-induced cardiomyopathy [35], and reviewed in many papers [26, 39, 40, 48]. It has established itself as a marker of myocardial tissue characterization, particularly as it relates to diffuse interstitial and infiltrative interstitial fibrosis.

Population Studies

Multi-Ethnic Study of Atherosclerosis (MESA) study is a prospective, population-based, epidemiologic study, which started in 2000 to investigate the prevalence and progression of subclinical cardiovascular disease in a multiethnic cohort (white, black, Hispanic, and Chinese). T1 mapping was included as part of the imaging protocol in the fifth follow-up examination of the MESA study, allowing for characterization of T1 mapping indices at the population level in a well-phenotyped cohort groups. Liu et al. [41] reported the T1 mapping parameters, which have been associated with myocardial fibrosis related to aging process. A total of 1231 study participants (51% women; age range 54–93 years) of the MESA cohort were evaluated with T1 mapping by using 1.5-T CMR scanners.

Women had significantly greater partition coefficient, ECV, and pre-contrast T1 than men, as well as lower post-contrast T1 values (all $p < 0.05$).

Linear regression analyses demonstrated that greater partition coefficient, pre-contrast T1 values, and ECV were associated with older age in men (multivariate regression coefficients = 0.01; 5.9 ms; and 1.04% per 10 years' change; all $p < 0.05$) [41]. Therefore, even though women had higher baseline ECV than men, they had lower increase in ECV over time. This study demonstrates the importance of considering age and sex while interpreting values from T1 mapping.

Donekal et al. assessed 1116 subjects who participated in the MESA study without an LGE-defined myocardial scar. They reported that there were sex-specific differences in diffuse interstitial fibrosis associated with cardiac remodeling. They observed that with increased extracellular matrix expansion, both men and women have reduced circumferential shortening as well as left ventricular end-diastolic mass and volume. In addition, lower post-contrast T1 times were associated with lower early diastolic strain rate in women only, and lower LV torsion and lower LV ejection fraction in men only [42]. Additionally, Ambale-Venkatesh et al. showed that an increasingly concentric pattern of remodeling was associated with diffuse interstitial fibrosis. In male subjects, this was also associated with a longitudinal decrease in ejection fraction [49]. Taken together, these studies highlight the impact of diffuse interstitial fibrosis on myocardial structure and function.

STEMI [45, 46]

Reinstadler et al. conducted native T1 mapping of 255 patients with re-vascularized STEMI with on days 2–5 and at 6 months follow-up.

Assessment of remote zone alterations by quantitative non-contrast T1-mapping showed a strong association with future major adverse cardiovascular events (MACE, T1 values >1129 ms; AUC 0.78; 95% CI 0.70–0.86; $p < 0.001$)) [45].

Biesbroek et al. investigated 42 native T1 and ECV of remote myocardium after AMI and explored their relation to left ventricular (LV) remodeling. They found ECV of remote myocardium decreased over time (3 months) in patients with no LV dilatation but remained elevated at follow-up in those who developed LV dilatation. (30 ± 2.0 vs. $27 \pm 2.3\%$, $p = 0.03$) [46].

These studies highlight the prognostic potential of assessment of both inflammation/edema and diffuse interstitial fibrosis using native T1 and ECV measures in STEMI participants.

Non-ischemic Heart Disease

Diastolic Cardiomyopathy (DCM) [34, 47]

Puntmann et al. investigated the use of T1 mapping to predict outcome in DCM patients in a prospective, observational, multi-center longitudinal study in 637 consecutive patients with non-ischemic dilated cardiomyopathy (NIDCM, median follow-up period of 22 months).

Among the deceased 28 patients, 50% showed positive LGE, while among the 609 survivors, 26% patients had positive LGE ($p = 0.005$). LGE was effective to identify high risk DCM patients, though in several patients with a diagnosis of DCM, LGE was negative.

In univariate Cox regression analysis, native T1 and LGE extent were the independent predictor variables in prediction of the outcome endpoints for all-cause mortality. (For native T1 per 10 ms change, hazard ratio 1.1; 95% CI 1.05–1.1; $p < 0.001$, for LGE extent, hazard ratio 1.09; 95% CI 1.02–1.16; $p = 0.009$.) For HF endpoint, native T1 was the independent predictor (hazard ratio 1.07; 95% CI 1.04–1.1; $p < 0.001$), while LGE was not. Predictive associations of T1 mapping indices were notably stronger compared to LGE for the HF endpoint. The authors discussed that unlike fixed, irreversible injury seen by LGE, the activity of diffuse disease detected by T1 mapping portrays the compensatory capacity within the remaining viable myocardium. T1 mapping may have potential to assess not only the histological change of the myocardium, but also its reversibility or capacity to react to the treatment [34]. T1 mapping, in addition to identifying area of necrosis (also highlighted in LGE), may be highlighting areas of injury and intracellular inflammation.

Youn et al. have reported from their single-center, prospective, cohort study of 117 NIDCM patients (71 men, 51.9 ± 16.7 years) who underwent clinical 3.0-T CMR that ECV increase (per 3%) was associated with a hazard ratio of 1.80 (95% confidence interval [CI], 1.48–2.20; $p < 0.001$) for MACE. Multivariable analysis also indicated that ECV was an independent prognostic factor (Harrell's c statistic, 0.88) than LGE quantification values (0.77) or mid-wall LGE (0.80) [47].

These two studies showed stronger prognostic capability of T1 mapping, over and above that of LGE in DCM patients. T1 mapping is already a clinically recommended tool for use in DCM. T1 mapping provides an important tool to treat and diagnose DCM.

Anthracycline-Induced Cardiomyopathy [35]

Neilan et al. have measured ECV in 42 adult patients treated with anthracyclines and compared them to healthy volunteers. The anthracycline group was all LGE negative. However, the ECV was elevated in the anthracycline-treated patients compared to the age- and gender-matched controls (0.36–0.03 vs. 0.28–0.02, $p < 0.001$). In addition, ECV was associated with worse diastolic function and increased atrial volumes.

LGE in anthracycline-induced cardiomyopathy is negative in a large proportion of participants as seen in the previous reports. T1 mapping, particularly in this category of patients, has strong potential to assess the diffuse fibrosis known as the late-toxicity following anthracycline therapy.

T1 Mapping in Stem Cell Therapy

The Rationale of T1 Mapping in the Study of Stem Cell Therapy

Stem cell therapy represents a novel approach, which has promised to restore the cardiac dysfunction and allow better prognosis. Previous clinical studies have presented inconsistent results but those could be because of the inappropriate expectation of LVEF recovery or reduced sensitivity to small reductions in LGE. In stem cell therapy, detection of subtle changes in both in cardiac function or myocardial morphology may be required. For the assessment of cardiac function, systolic and diastolic deformation as well as torsion are being considered as alternate parameters. For the assessment of myocardial tissue characteristics, T1 mapping may be a promising technique to detect diffuse fibrosis as well as subtle changes in the properties of the scar and peri-infarct regions. The use of T1 mapping in stem cell therapy may help us localize therapeutic benefits to the areas of scar, gray zone or remote myocardium. Such information may be useful for not only quantifying the magnitude of therapeutic effects but also in understanding the underlying mechanisms and reduction of MACE—eventually leading to more effective and appropriate interventional strategies.

The prognostic ability of T1 mapping is another compelling reason to assess the patients undergoing cell therapy. In some DCM studies, the prognostic prediction was more reliable than LGE [34, 47]. Longitudinal changes in T1 mapping may contribute to assess the patients' prognosis and lead to modification of management plan. T1 mapping studies, which assessed the disease characteristics and provided prognostic data need further investigation to confirm the longitudinal changes based on the extent of changes in ECV and T1-map over wide range of follow-up durations.

It is important to choose suitable T1 mapping indices when assessing the efficacy of stem cell therapy in patients. Pre-contrast T1 (Native T1) measures the T1 values from the composite of extracellular and intracellular compartments while post-contrast T1 derived ECV assesses extracellular expansion. With stem cell therapy, likely effects include decreased extracellular fibrosis, reduced inflammation/hypertrophy as well as myocyte regeneration and/or preservation. While reduction in myocardial fibrosis, is linked to reduction in extracellular space, and reflected in ECV reduction, changes in myocyte integrity as well as inflammation are also expected to reduce the ECV. Taken together, we expect the effect of stem cell therapy will drive to reduce ECV and shorten the native T1.

In conclusion, we report that there is significant rationale to employ T1 mapping and conventional, well-investigated technique of LGE in assessing the clinical benefit of stem cell therapy. Precise assessment of myocardial fibrosis, inflammation, and ECV changes will enable sensitive assessment of cardiac parameters including, diastolic function, torsion, and strain in stem cell therapy. These novel measurements will complement the traditional evaluation of LVEF and ventricular volumes.

References

1. Chiu RC, Zibaitis A, Kao RL. Cellular cardiomyoplasty: myocardial regeneration with satellite cell implantation. Ann Thorac Surg. 1995;60:12–8.
2. Perin EC, Dohmann HFR, Borojevic R, et al. Transendocardial, autologous bone marrow cell transplantation for severe, chronic ischemic heart failure. Circulation. 2003;107(18):2294–302. https://doi.org/10.1161/01.CIR.0000070596.30552.8B.
3. Psaltis PJ, Zannettino ACW, Gronthos S, Worthley SG. Intramyocardial navigation and mapping for stem cell delivery. J Cardiovasc Transl Res. 2010;3:135–46.
4. Wollert KC, Meyer GP, Lotz J, et al. Intracoronary autologous bone-marrow cell transfer after myocardial infarction: the BOOST randomised controlled clinical trial. Lancet. 2004;364:141–8.
5. Lunde K, Solheim S, Aakhus S, et al. Intracoronary injection of mononuclear bone marrow cells in acute myocardial infarction. N Engl J Med. 2006;355:1199–209.
6. Hirsch A, Nijveldt R, van der Vleuten PA, et al. Intracoronary infusion of mononuclear cells from bone marrow or peripheral blood compared with standard therapy in patients after acute myocardial infarction treated by primary percutaneous coronary intervention: results of the randomized controlled HEBE. Eur Heart J. 2011;32:1736–47.
7. Malliaras K, Makkar RR, Smith RR, et al. Intracoronary cardiosphere-derived cells after myocardial infarction: evidence of therapeutic regeneration in the final 1-year results of the CADUCEUS trial (CArdiosphere-Derived aUtologous stem CElls to reverse ventricUlar dySfunction). J Am Coll Cardiol. 2014;63:110–22.
8. Bolli R, Chugh AR, D'Amario D, et al. Cardiac stem cells in patients with ischaemic cardiomyopathy (SCIPIO): initial results of a randomised phase 1 trial. Lancet (London, England). 2011;378:1847–57.
9. Heldman AW, DiFede DL, Fishman JE, et al. Transendocardial mesenchymal stem cells and mononuclear bone marrow cells for ischemic cardiomyopathy: the TAC-HFT randomized trial. JAMA. 2014;311:62–73.
10. Fischer-Rasokat U, Assmus B, Seeger FH, et al. A pilot trial to assess potential effects of selective intracoronary bone marrow-derived progenitor cell infusion in patients with nonischemic dilated cardiomyopathy: final 1-year results of the transplantation of progenitor cells and functional regenerat. Circ Heart Fail. 2009;2:417–23.
11. Seth S, Bhargava B, Narang R, Ray R, Mohanty S, Gulati G, Kumar L, Airan B, Venugopal P, AIIMS Stem Cell Study Group. The ABCD (Autologous Bone Marrow Cells in Dilated Cardiomyopathy) trial a long-term follow-up study. J Am Coll Cardiol. 2010;55:1643–4.
12. Vrtovec B, Poglajen G, Lezaic L, Sever M, Socan A, Domanovic D, Cernelc P, Torre-Amione G, Haddad F, Wu JC. Comparison of transendocardial and intracoronary CD34+ cell transplantation in patients with nonischemic dilated cardiomyopathy. Circulation. 2013;128:S42–9.
13. Hare JM, DiFede DL, Rieger AC, et al. Randomized comparison of allogeneic versus autologous mesenchymal stem cells for nonischemic dilated cardiomyopathy. J Am Coll Cardiol. 2017;69:526–37.
14. Lee J-W, Lee S-H, Youn Y-J, et al. A randomized, open-label, multicenter trial for the safety and efficacy of adult mesenchymal stem cells after acute myocardial infarction. J Korean Med Sci. 2014;29:23.
15. Madonna R, Van Laake LW, Davidson SM, et al. Position paper of the European Society of Cardiology Working Group cellular biology of the heart: cell-based therapies for myocardial repair and regeneration in ischemic heart disease and heart failure. Eur Heart J. 2016;37:1789–98.
16. Hare JM, Fishman JE, Gerstenblith G, et al. Comparison of allogeneic vs autologous bone marrow–derived mesenchymal stem cells delivered by transendocardial injection in patients with ischemic cardiomyopathy. JAMA. 2012;308:2369.
17. Charoenpanichkit C, Hundley W. The 20 year evolution of dobutamine stress cardiovascular magnetic resonance. J Cardiovasc Magn Reson. 2010;12:59.
18. Meyer GP, Wollert KC, Lotz J, et al. Intracoronary bone marrow cell transfer after myocardial infarction: eighteen months' follow-up data from the

randomized, controlled BOOST (Bone marrow transfer to enhance ST-elevation infarct regeneration) trial. Circulation. 2006;113:1287–94.

19. Fisher SA, Zhang H, Doree C, Mathur A, Martin-Rendon E. Stem cell treatment for acute myocardial infarction. Cochrane Database Syst Rev. 2015;(2):CD006536.

20. Afzal MR, Samanta A, Shah ZI, Jeevanantham V, Abdel-Latif A, Zuba-Surma EK, Dawn B. Adult bone marrow cell therapy for ischemic heart disease: evidence and insights from randomized controlled trials. Circ Res. 2015;117:558–75.

21. Henry TD, Moyé L, Traverse JH. Consistently inconsistent-bone marrow mononuclear stem cell therapy following acute myocardial infarction: a decade later. Circ Res. 2016;119.404 6.

22. Suerder D, Manka R, Moccetti T, et al. The effect of bone marrow derived mononuclear cell treatment, early or late after acute myocardial infarction: twelve months CMR and long-term clinical results. Circ Res. 2016;119(3):481–90. https://doi.org/10.1161/CIRCRESAHA.116.308639.

23. Solomon SD, Anavekar N, Skali H, et al. Influence of ejection fraction on cardiovascular outcomes in a broad spectrum of heart failure patients. Circulation. 2005;112:3738–44.

24. Hsu JJ, Ziaeian B, Fonarow GC. Heart failure with mid-range (borderline) ejection fraction. JACC Hear Fail. 2017;5:763–71.

25. Yan AT, Shayne AJ, Brown KA, Gupta SN, Chan CW, Luu TM, Di Carli MF, Reynolds HG, Stevenson WG, Kwong RY. Characterization of the peri-infarct zone by contrast-enhanced cardiac magnetic resonance imaging is a powerful predictor of post-myocardial infarction mortality. Circulation. 2006;114:32–9.

26. Avelar E, Strickland CR, Rosito G. Role of imaging in cardio-oncology. Curr Treat Options Cardiovasc Med. 2017;19(6):46. https://doi.org/10.1007/s11936-017-0546-2.

27. Kim RJ, Wu E, Rafael A, Chen EL, Parker MA, Simonetti O, Klocke FJ, Bonow RO, Judd RM. The use of contrast-enhanced magnetic resonance imaging to identify reversible myocardial dysfunction. N Engl J Med. 2000;343:1445–53.

28. Hamirani YS, Wong A, Kramer CM, Salerno M. Effect of microvascular obstruction and intramyocardial hemorrhage by CMR on LV remodeling and outcomes after myocardial infarction: a systematic review and meta-analysis. JACC Cardiovasc Imaging. 2014;7:940–52.

29. Gulati A, Jabbour A, Ismail TF, et al. Association of fibrosis with mortality and sudden cardiac death in patients with nonischemic dilated cardiomyopathy. JAMA. 2013;309:896–908.

30. Assomull RG, Prasad SK, Lyne J, Smith G, Burman ED, Khan M, Sheppard MN, Poole-Wilson PA, Pennell DJ. Cardiovascular magnetic resonance, fibrosis, and prognosis in dilated cardiomyopathy. J Am Coll Cardiol. 2006;48:1977–85.

31. Bruder O, Wagner A, Jensen CJ, et al. Myocardial scar visualized by cardiovascular magnetic resonance imaging predicts major adverse events in patients with hypertrophic cardiomyopathy. J Am Coll Cardiol. 2010;56:875–87.

32. Greulich S, Deluigi CC, Gloekler S, et al. CMR imaging predicts death and other adverse events in suspected cardiac sarcoidosis. JACC Cardiovasc Imaging. 2013;6:501–11.

33. Mahrholdt H, Wagner A, Judd RM, Sechtem U, Kim RJ. Delayed enhancement cardiovascular magnetic resonance assessment of non-ischaemic cardiomyopathies. Eur Heart J. 2005;26:1461–74.

34. Puntmann VO, Carr-White G, Jabbour A, et al. T1-mapping and outcome in nonischemic cardiomyopathy. JACC Cardiovasc Imaging. 2016;9:40–50.

35. Neilan TG, Coelho Filho OR, Shah RV, et al. Myocardial extracellular volume by cardiac magnetic resonance imaging in patients treated with anthracycline-based chemotherapy. Am J Cardiol. 2013;111:717–22.

36. Ambale-Venkatesh B, Lima JAC. Cardiac MRI: a central prognostic tool in myocardial fibrosis. Nat Rev Cardiol. 2015;12:18–29.

37. Mewton N, Liu CY, Croisille P, Bluemke D, Lima JAC. Assessment of myocardial fibrosis with cardiovascular magnetic resonance. J Am Coll Cardiol. 2011;57:891–903.

38. Maestrini V, Treibel TA, White SK, Fontana M, Moon JC. T1 mapping for characterization of intracellular and extracellular myocardial diseases in heart failure. Curr Cardiovasc Imaging Rep. 2014;7:1–7.

39. Puntmann VO, Peker E, Chandrashekhar Y, Nagel E. T1 mapping in characterizing myocardial disease: a comprehensive review. Circ Res. 2016;119:277–99.

40. Haaf P, Garg P, Messroghli DR, Broadbent DA, Greenwood JP, Plein S. Cardiac T1 mapping and extracellular volume (ECV) in clinical practice: a comprehensive review. J Cardiovasc Magn Reson. 2017;18:89.

41. Liu C-Y, Liu Y-C, Wu C, et al. Evaluation of age-related interstitial myocardial fibrosis with cardiac magnetic resonance contrast-enhanced T1 mapping: MESA (Multi-Ethnic Study of Atherosclerosis). J Am Coll Cardiol. 2013;62:1280–7.

42. Donekal S, Venkatesh BA, Liu YC, et al. Interstitial fibrosis, left ventricular remodeling, and myocardial mechanical behavior in a population-based multiethnic cohort: the multi-ethnic study of atherosclerosis (mesa) study. Circ Cardiovasc Imaging. 2014;7:292–302.

43. Inoue YY, Ambale-Venkatesh B, Mewton N, et al. Electrocardiographic impact of myocardial diffuse fibrosis and scar: MESA (Multi-Ethnic Study of Atherosclerosis). Radiology. 2017;282:690–8.

44. Yi CJ, Wu CO, Tee M, et al. The association between cardiovascular risk and cardiovascular magnetic resonance measures of fibrosis: the Multi-Ethnic Study of Atherosclerosis (MESA). J Cardiovasc Magn Reson. 2015;17(1):15.

45. Reinstadler SJ, Stiermaier T, Liebetrau J, et al. 9Prognostic significance of remote myocardium alterations assessed by quantitative noncontrast T1 mapping in ST-segment elevation myocardial infarction. JACC Cardiovasc Imaging. 2017;11(3):411–9. https://doi.org/10.1016/j.jcmg.2017.03.015.

46. Biesbroek PS, Amier RP, Teunissen PFA, Hofman MBM, Robbers LFHJ, van de Ven PM, Beek AM, van Rossum AC, van Royen N, Nijveldt R. Changes in remote myocardial tissue after acute myocardial infarction and its relation to cardiac remodeling: a CMR T1 mapping study. PLoS One. 2017;12:1–13.

47. Youn J-C, Hong YJ, Lee H-J, et al. Contrast-enhanced T1 mapping-based extracellular volume fraction independently predicts clinical outcome in patients with non-ischemic dilated cardiomyopathy: a prospective cohort study. Eur Radiol. 2017;27(9):3924–33. https://doi.org/10.1007/s00330-017-4817-9.

48. Hamdy A, Kitagawa K, Ishida M, Sakuma H. Native myocardial T1 mapping, are we there yet? Int Heart J. 2016;57:400–7.

49. Venkatesh BA, Volpe GJ, Donekal S, et al. Association of longitudinal changes in left ventricular structure and function with myocardial fibrosis: the Multi-Ethnic Study of Atherosclerosis study. Hypertension. 2014;64:508–15.

T1 Mapping in Uncommon Non-ischemic Cardiomyopathies

Kate Hanneman

Introduction

Non-ischemic cardiomyopathy (NICM) is a broad term that refers to diseases affecting the myocardium other than atherosclerosis. NICM encompasses myocardial diseases associated with mechanical or electrical dysfunction exhibiting inappropriate ventricular hypertrophy or dilatation. The causes are numerous, but an increasing number of non-ischemic disorders are being recognized as genetic in cause [1].

Cardiac magnetic resonance (CMR) has a unique role in the evaluation of NICM, including the ability to add information regarding tissue composition. CMR enables accurate measurement of left ventricular (LV) volumes, mass, and ejection fraction. Late gadolinium enhancement (LGE) is useful in differentiating ischemic cardiomyopathy from NICM, and distinguishing between different types of NICM based upon the pattern and distribution of enhancement [2]. LGE identifies replacement myocardial fibrosis, which has diagnostic [3] and prognostic [4] value, although it is usually irreversible. A potential pitfall of LGE is that it may fail to characterize diffuse interstitial myocardial fibrosis due to reliance on relative signal intensity changes [5].

Recent advances in CMR allow for quantification of the myocardial longitudinal relaxation time constant (T1) using a single, short breath-hold mapping sequence. T1 is an intrinsic magnetic property of tissue that represents longitudinal recovery time of hydrogen atoms after excitation. Each tissue has its own characteristic range of T1 values, which may be altered in disease. Deviation from normal tissue-specific T1 values is used to quantify the effects of pathological processes. Some pathologies, including fat, iron, and amyloid, change T1 substantially, while others have smaller effects. T1 maps can be produced of non-contrast myocardial T1 values or post-contrast myocardial T1 values after administration of gadolinium-based contrast [6]. The combination of pre- and post-contrast T1 mapping allows for assessment of the myocardial partition coefficient, lambda, with subsequent derivation of the extracellular volume (ECV) fraction by adjustment for the contrast distribution volume.

A potential benefit of T1 mapping over LGE techniques, is that administration of contrast is not required. This is important in the subset of patients who have concomitant renal dysfunction precluding safe administration of gadolinium-based contrast agents, which are necessary for LGE imaging. Impaired renal function is a concern particularly in the setting of advanced amyloidosis and Fabry disease. In this setting, administration of gadolinium based contrast places the patient at a theoretical risk of nephrogenic systemic

K. Hanneman, MD, MPH, FRCPC
Department of Medical Imaging, Toronto General Hospital, University of Toronto, Toronto, ON, Canada
e-mail: kate.hanneman@uhn.ca

sclerosis (NSF). T1 mapping also allows for quantification, potentially standardizing CMR measurements of myocardial tissue properties.

Multiple different T1 mapping techniques are currently employed, including modified Look–Locker inversion recovery (MOLLI), shortened MOLLI sequence (ShMOLLI), saturation recovery single-shot acquisition (SASHA), and saturation pulse prepared heart-rate-independent inversion recovery (SAPPHIRE) techniques. MOLLI and ShMOLLI systematically underestimate native myocardial T1 in comparison to standard spin echo acquisition, whereas SASHA and SAPPHIRE yield higher accuracy but lower precision compared with MOLLI and ShMOLLI for T1 measurements [7]. T1 values also vary with multiple other parameters, including the magnetic field strength, with significantly higher values at 3T compared to 1.5T. This means that different techniques measure different normal values, and, therefore, T1 measurements must be interpreted based on the specific technique employed.

Non-contrast myocardial T1 values are elevated, post-contrast T1 values are reduced, and ECV values are elevated when the extra-cellular space is expanded, such as in the setting of myocardial fibrosis. Increased ECV has been shown to correlate with histologic measures of fibrosis [8]. However, not all alterations in T1 and ECV values reflect myocardial fibrosis. Increased non-contrast T1 and ECV values have also been described in the setting of cardiac amyloid infiltration, which also results in expansion of the extra-cellular space. Myocardial edema, which can be present in the setting of acute inflammation and myocarditis, also results in elevated non-contrast T1 and ECV values. Therefore, non-contrast myocardial T1 and ECV values are expected to be elevated in the setting of fibrosis, infarct, edema and amyloid [9–11]. On the other hand, non-contrast T1 values have been shown to be reduced in several conditions including iron overload, fat infiltration, Fabry disease and hemorrhage [12–14]. Myocardial T1 and ECV values must be interpreted within the context of clinical and other imaging data.

This chapter will discuss the role of CMR T1 mapping in the evaluation of less common NICMs including Anderson-Fabry (Fabry) disease, iron overload, amyloidosis, and sarcoidosis, highlighting the potential role of T1 mapping beyond assessment of myocardial fibrosis.

Fabry Disease

Fabry disease is a rare, X-linked inherited disorder of lysosomal metabolism caused by reduced or absent activity of the alpha galactosidase enzyme, resulting in lysosomal sphingolipid accumulation in a number of different organs including the heart [15]. Since the introduction of renal replacement therapy, the main cause of mortality in Fabry disease is cardiac disease. Left ventricular hypertrophy (LVH), valve thickening, myocardial scarring, heart failure and sudden arrhythmic death can occur [16]. Patients with Fabry disease can be treated with enzyme replacement therapy, which should be initiated before reversible end-organ damage has occurred [17].

Classic CMR findings in Fabry disease include concentric LVH and midwall LGE involving the basal inferolateral segment [18]. However, this classic imaging phenotype is only seen in a minority of patients [19]. Distinguishing Fabry-related LVH from other causes of LVH remains a major clinical and imaging challenge.

In Fabry disease, non-contrast T1 values are substantially lower compared to healthy controls and to patients with other causes of LVH including aortic stenosis and hypertrophic cardiomyopathy (HCM) [20, 21]. In patients with LVH, non-contrast T1 values discriminate between Fabry disease and other diseases causing LVH with no overlap [20]. Even in patients without LVH, non-contrast T1 values are reduced compared to normal controls, and are associated with reduced echocardiographic-based global longitudinal speckle tracking strain and early diastolic function impairment [14]. Mean non-contrast T1 values in Fabry disease have been reported at 853 ms in patients without LVH (ShMOLLI at 1.5T) [14], 882–904 ms in patients with LVH (ShMOLLI at 1.5T) [14, 20], and 1053–1096 ms using a different technique (SASHA at 1.5T) [21, 22]. However, there is no significant difference in myocardial ECV values between patients with Fabry disease and healthy controls [21, 23]. An example of T1 mapping in a patient with Fabry disease is shown in Fig. 8.1.

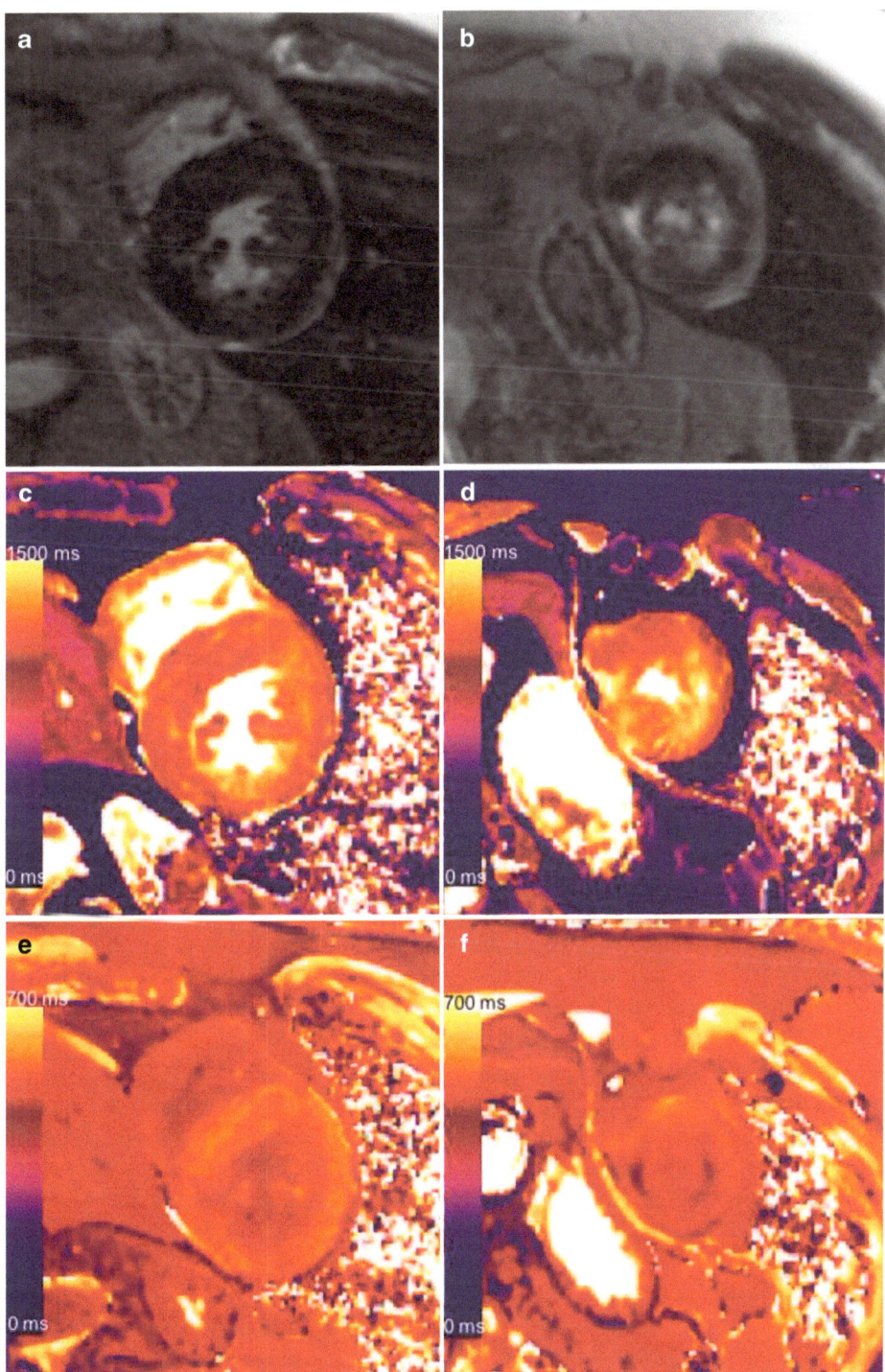

Fig. 8.1 53-year-old male with Fabry disease. There is concentric left ventricular (LV) hypertrophy and elevated LV mass (LV mass indexed to BSA 154.9 g/m²). Short axis mid (**a**) and apical (**b**) late gadolinium enhanced (LGE) images demonstrated mid wall LGE in the apical segments, which is not typical of Fabry disease. Short axis mid (**c**) and apical (**d**) non-contrast T1 maps (MOLLI, 3T) demonstrate mildly reduced T1 values (mean 1030 ms) in non-LGE areas, and pseudonormalization of T1 values (mean 1150 ms) in LGE-positive areas. Short axis mid (**e**) and apical (**f**) post-contrast T1 maps demonstrate mean myocardial post-contrast T1 value of 465 ms

Reduced non-contrast myocardial T1 values in Fabry disease may be the consequence of increased glycosphingolipid concentration in the myocardium. Lipids have characteristically lower T1 values, approximately 250 ms at 1.5T, which would result in a reduction in the apparent tissue T1 values. In a small sample of patients with Fabry disease, single-voxel NMR spectroscopy demonstrated a significant negative linear relationship between lipid content and non-contrast T1 values, suggesting that non-contrast T1 may be directly measuring myocardial storage [21]. This is supported by pathology results demonstrating relatively high myocardial concentrations of the glycolipid ceramide trihexoside in patients with Fabry disease [24]. Water constraint and water-lipid and water-protein interactions have been shown to cause T1 lowering in myelin, rather than a direct signal from lipid protons, and these mechanisms may also contribute to the non-contrast T1 decrease seen in Fabry disease [20].

Focal fibrosis in the basal inferolateral wall has been previously documented in Fabry disease using LGE [18]. Non-contrast T1 values demonstrate pseudonormalization or elevation of T1 in the left ventricular inferolateral wall if LGE is present, potentially allowing for identification of focal fibrosis without the need for contrast administration [20].

Compared to males, females with Fabry disease have lower LV mass and wall thickness, higher non-contrast myocardial T1 values and higher ECV [21]. Although Fabry disease is an X-linked disease, female carriers also exhibit significant heart disease and genetic testing is currently recommended for the diagnosis of Fabry disease in women, highlighting a potential role of T1 mapping for noninvasive diagnosis and monitoring in both sexes [25].

Iron Overload

Lifelong blood transfusions and altered iron homeostasis frequently result in multi-organ iron overload in patients with thalassemia major and other hematologic anemias. Myocardial iron overload confers a poor prognosis with heart failure

and arrhythmia as the major causes of death [26]. Timely implementation of adequate iron chelation therapy prevents further cardiac dysfunction and improves survival. However, once heart failure develops, the prognosis is usually poor. Iron chelation therapy is effective but has side effects and is costly, therefore, treatment needs to be initiated and tailored based on individual need.

CMR is well established in the evaluation and management of patients with transfusion dependent anemias. Iron is paramagnetic, causing inhomogeneity within the local magnetic field, and results in shortening of all three fundamental tissue signal MRI rate constants: T1, T2, and T2* [27, 28]. CMR T2* imaging has been validated histologically in severe iron overload and has high sensitivity, reproducibility and prognostic value [28–30]. Cardiac iron concentration is inversely related to myocardial T2* values [27]. There has been significant improvement in the survival of patients with cardiac iron overload subsequent to the introduction of the CMR T2* imaging [31]. However, there are limitations to CMR T2* analysis, including the need for a long breath-hold, susceptibility artifacts more pronounced at 3T compared to 1.5T, and reduced discrimination in both early and very severe iron overload [32].

As iron interacts with water protons, it affects the T1 relaxation time. T1 has been shown to change with tissue iron in a gerbil iron overload model but with smaller effect relative to T2 and T2* changes [33]. Studies in humans have demonstrated that myocardial T1 values correlate positively with T2* values [11, 34, 35]. T1 mapping may be more sensitive and reproducible than T2* in the detection of myocardial iron [11, 36]. Myocardial ECV is significantly elevated in thalassemia major and is associated with iron overload [35]. In patients with myocardial iron overload, reported mean T1 values are 474–804 ms at 1.5T (MOLLI) and 653–1056 ms at 3T (MOLLI) [34, 36, 37]. An example of T2* and T1 mapping in a patient with iron overload is shown in Fig. 8.2. An example of T2* and T1 mapping in a patient without iron overload is shown in Fig. 8.3.

T1 mapping may be particularly useful in the setting of very severe iron overload and mild iron

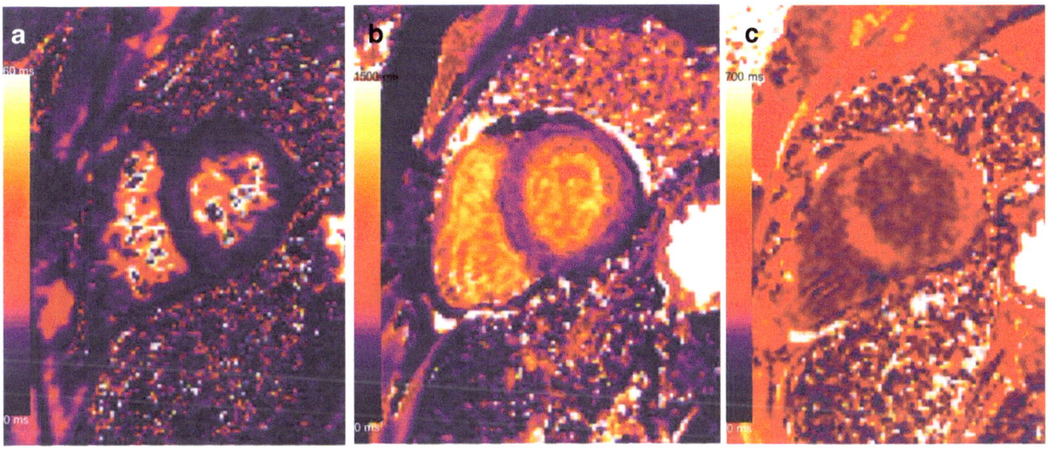

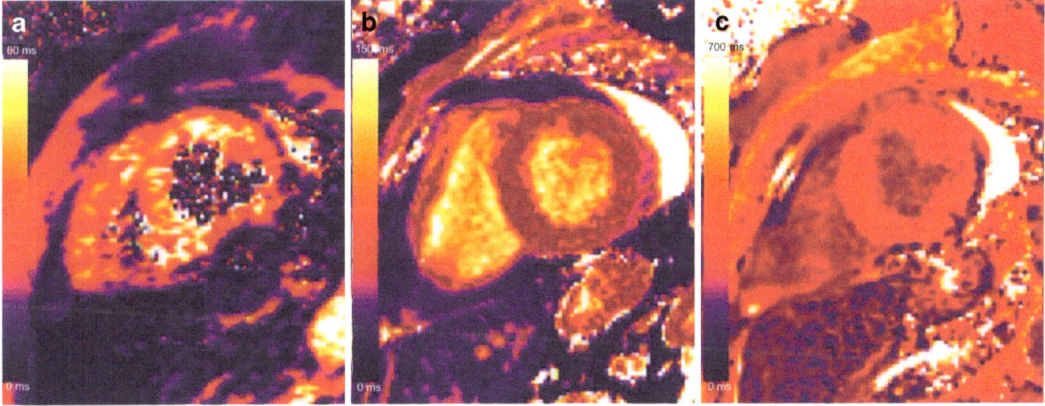

Fig. 8.2 29-year-old transfusion dependent female with beta-thalassemia major. Basal short-axis T2* map (**a**) demonstrates a mean septal T2* value of 8 ms, consistent with severe iron overload. Basal short-axis non-contrast T1 map (**b**) demonstrates reduced T1 value (mean 690 ms, MOLLI, 1.5T), consistent with the presence of myocardial iron. Basal short-axis post-contrast T1 map (**c**) demonstrates a mean T1 value of 274 ms. Global myocardial ECV was calculated at 32%

Fig. 8.3 45-year-old transfusion dependent male with beta-thalassemia major, treated with chelation therapy. Mid-ventricular short-axis T2* map (**a**) demonstrates a mean septal T2* value of 38 ms, within the normal range, with no evidence of myocardial iron overload. Mid short-axis non-contrast T1 map (**b**) demonstrates a mean T1 value of 961 ms (MOLLI, 1.5T). Mid short-axis post-contrast T1 map (**c**) demonstrates a mean T1 value of 377 ms. Global myocardial ECV was calculated at 33%

overload where T2* analysis should be used with caution as other factors affecting field homogeneity are important.

Amyloid

Amyloidosis refers to a family of diseases induced by misfolded or misassembled proteins. Several types of amyloid can involve the heart, including light-chain amyloidosis (AL) and transthyretin amyloidosis (ATTR) [38]. Cardiac involvement is most common with type AL amyloidosis, which is often associated with multiple myeloma or other monoclonal gammopathies. Cardiac amyloid has a very poor prognosis with progressive loss of ventricular compliance, diastolic dysfunction, and reduced systolic function, resulting in a restrictive cardiomyopathy. Treatment is dictated by the type and degree of cardiac involvement. Consequently, early recognition and accurate classification are essential.

Endomyocardial biopsy is the gold standard for diagnosing cardiac amyloidosis. However, it is invasive and prone to false negatives. Noninvasive tools for establishing a diagnosis of cardiac involvement include ECG, echocardiography, and CMR. ECG findings, including low QRS voltages, have low specificity, and echocardiography findings often become abnormal only late in the disease once patients are already symptomatic [39]. CMR markers of cardiac amyloid include increased left ventricular mass and wall thickness, abnormal nulling of myocardium on the cardiac MRI inversion scout (TI-scout) sequence, and diffuse late gadolinium enhancement most prominent in the subendocardium [40, 41]. The classic pattern of LGE matches the distribution of amyloid on histology. However, this characteristic pattern of LGE may only occur late in the disease process and does not quantify disease burden. In cases of diffuse myocardial involvement, the lack of a normal region of myocardium for comparison can make LGE images difficult to interpret. Finally, many patients with suspected cardiac amyloidosis have significant renal impairment making administration of gadolinium-based contrast problematic.

Amyloid AL patients with cardiac involvement have significantly elevated non-contrast T1 values compared to patients with aortic stenosis, with a similar degree of ventricular wall thickening [42]. A non-contrast T1 threshold of 1020 ms (ShMOLLI at 1.5T) resulted in 92% accuracy for diagnosis of cardiac amyloid [42]. Non-contrast T1 values are also significantly higher in patients with confirmed cardiac amyloid by immunohistochemistry of endomyocardial biopsy compared to patients with systemic amyloidosis without cardiac involvement [43]. Non-contrast T1 values correlate with markers of systolic and diastolic dysfunction, suggesting that elevated T1 values may reflect the severity of cardiac involvement [42]. T1 values are elevated not only in patients with definite cardiac involvement (1140 ms) but also in patients with possible (1048 ms) and no cardiac involvement (1009 ms) although at lower levels [42]. The pathophysiologic basis of the elevated T1 values in amyloid may be due to expansion of the interstitial space from fibrillar deposits. An example of T1 mapping in a patient with AL cardiac amyloid is shown in Fig. 8.4.

Non-contrast T1 values are also elevated in ATTR although values are not as high as in the AL subtype [44]. Average non-contrast T1 values in ATTR were 1097 ms compared with an average T1 value of 1130 ms in patients with AL amyloidosis (ShMOLLI at 1.5T). This difference may be clinically relevant because treatment and prognosis vary by subtype. An example of T1 mapping in a patient with ATTR cardiac amyloid is shown in Fig. 8.5.

Mean myocardial ECV is also significantly elevated in cardiac amyloidosis [45, 46]. Mean ECV has been shown to increase between groups from healthy controls (25.4%) to AL with no suspected cardiac involvement (27.6%), possible cardiac involvement (34.2%), and definite cardiac involvement (48.8%) [45].

Myocardial ECV and pre-contrast T1 values predict mortality in systemic AL amyloidosis. An ECV of 45% had a hazard ratio (HR) for death of 3.84, and a pre-contrast T1 value of 1044 ms had a HR of 5.39 (ShMOLLI at 1.5T) [46].

Non-contrast T1 and ECV values are elevated in cardiac amyloid and have prognostic significance. The ability to accurately identify cardiac amyloid and quantitatively assess the burden of disease without using contrast is a considerable advantage given the relatively high incidence of chronic kidney disease in this population.

Sarcoid

Sarcoidosis is a multi-system granulomatous disorder of unknown etiology, which can result in myocardial inflammation [47]. Development and accumulation of non-caseating granulomas are the pathologic hallmark of sarcoidosis, occurring most commonly within the pulmonary parenchyma and lymph nodes, but can involve many organ systems, including the heart [48]. Cardiac sarcoidosis may manifest clinically as a restrictive cardiomyopathy with complications including heart failure, arrhythmia, and sudden cardiac death

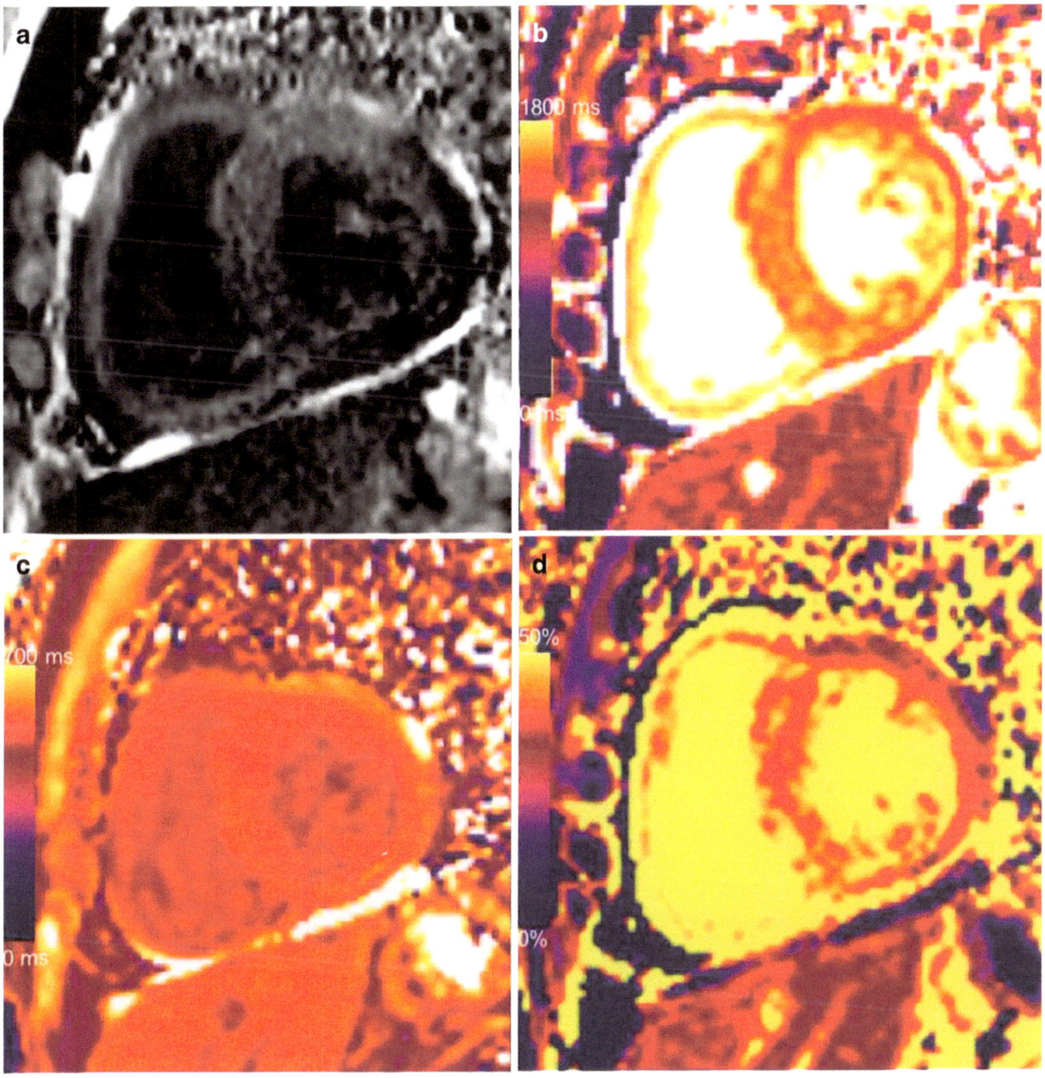

Fig. 8.4 60-year-old male with light chain (AL) cardiac amyloid confirmed with biopsy. Mid-ventricular short-axis PSIR image (**a**) demonstrates decreased signal intensity in the blood pool, diffuse myocardial enhancement typical of cardiac amyloid. Mid short-axis non-contrast T1 map (**b**) demonstrates diffusely elevated T1 values (mean 1443 ms) (MOLLI, 3T). Mid short-axis post-contrast T1 map (**c**) demonstrates a mean post-contrast T1 value of 450 ms. Mid short-axis ECV map (**d**) demonstrates elevated global myocardial ECV (mean 44%)

[47, 49]. Cardiac involvement accounts for up to 25% of disease-related deaths [50, 51].

The diagnosis of cardiac sarcoidosis remains challenging. Approximately 5% of patients with sarcoidosis have clinically apparent cardiac involvement, yet autopsy series indicate that cardiac involvement is present in up to 25% of cases [47, 51]. This discrepancy suggests that cardiac sarcoidosis is under-diagnosed in clinical practice. The diagnostic yield of endomyocardial biopsy is reported at less than 20% [52, 53].

Previous studies have demonstrated high diagnostic accuracy of both CMR [54–56] and 18F-labelled fluoro-2-deoxyglucose (FDG) PET [57, 58] for detection of cardiac sarcoid. CMR can identify myocardial inflammation and edema using T2-weighted imaging and macroscopic fibrosis using LGE [59–61]. In cardiac sarcoidosis, LGE may reflect accumulation of gadolinium chelate in tissue as a result of differences in the contrast distribution volume [52]. In the chronic phase, foci of LGE may reflect

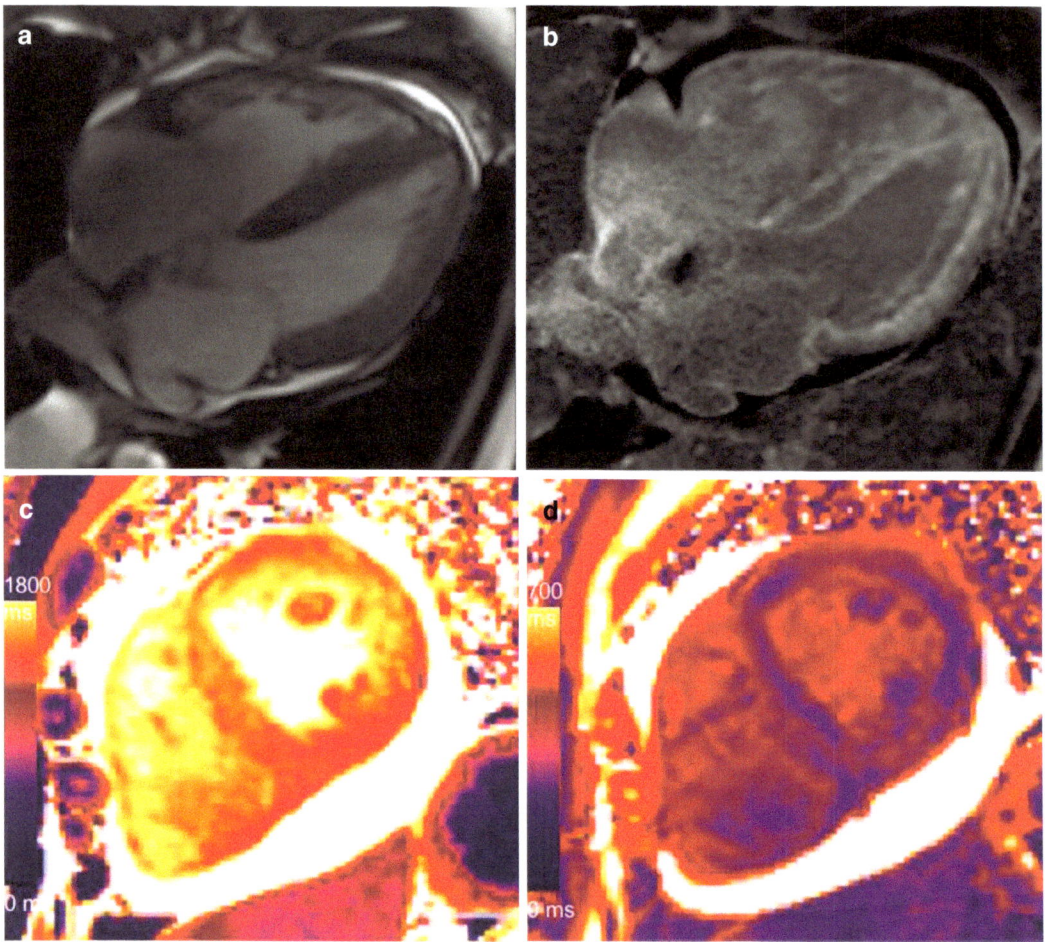

Fig. 8.5 61-year-old male with ATTR cardiac amyloid. Four-chamber cine SSFP image (**a**) demonstrates biatrial enlargement, small pericardial and pleural effusions, and concentric left ventricular hypertrophy. Four-chamber LGE image (**b**) demonstrates diffuse enhancement most prominent in the subendocardium and decreased signal intensity in the blood pool, typical of cardiac amyloid. Mid ventricular short-axis non-contrast T1 map (**c**) demonstrates diffusely elevated T1 values (mean 1340 ms, MOLLI, 3T). Mid short-axis post-contrast T1 map (**d**) demonstrates a mean T1 value of 330 ms

replacement fibrosis with increased interstitial concentration of contrast [62]. The pattern of LGE in cardiac sarcoidosis is typically patchy or nodular, and predominantly located in the mid wall and epicardium [52]. There is a growing body of evidence suggesting that the presence and extent of myocardial scar and interstitial fibrosis provides a substrate for ventricular arrhythmias [54, 63].

LGE MRI detects nonviable myocardium, but is less sensitive to inflamed but viable myocardium that occurs in the acute and potentially reversible early stages of cardiac sarcoidosis [64]. T2-weighted CMR has been successfully applied to detect myocardial edema in the setting of acute myocardial inflammation [65, 66], and has been shown to improve the detection of active myocarditis and cardiac sarcoidosis compared with LGE alone [67, 68].

No prospective studies have reported T1 mapping and ECV analysis in patients with cardiac sarcoidosis. However in acute myocarditis, non-contrast T1 mapping has been shown to have higher sensitivity compared with T2 weighted imaging and LGE techniques in detecting areas of myocardial inflammation and/or edema [69]. A threshold of T1 > 990 ms (sensitivity 90%, specificity 88%) detected significantly larger areas of involvement than T2W and LGE imaging in patients, and additional areas of injury when T2W and LGE were negative (ShMOLLI at 1.5T) [70]. Non-contrast T1-mapping displays the typical non-ischemic patterns in acute myocarditis similar to LGE imaging but without the need for contrast agents. Elevated non-contrast values suggestive of edema have also been reported in patients with systemic lupus erythematosus [71]. Given that myocardial edema and inflammation are characteristic features in the acute phase of cardiac sarcoid, T1 mapping may also be useful in this setting.

An example of T1 and T2 mapping in a patient with cardiac sarcoid is shown in Fig. 8.6. An example of T1 mapping in a patient with pulmonary sarcoid without cardiac involvement is shown in Fig. 8.7.

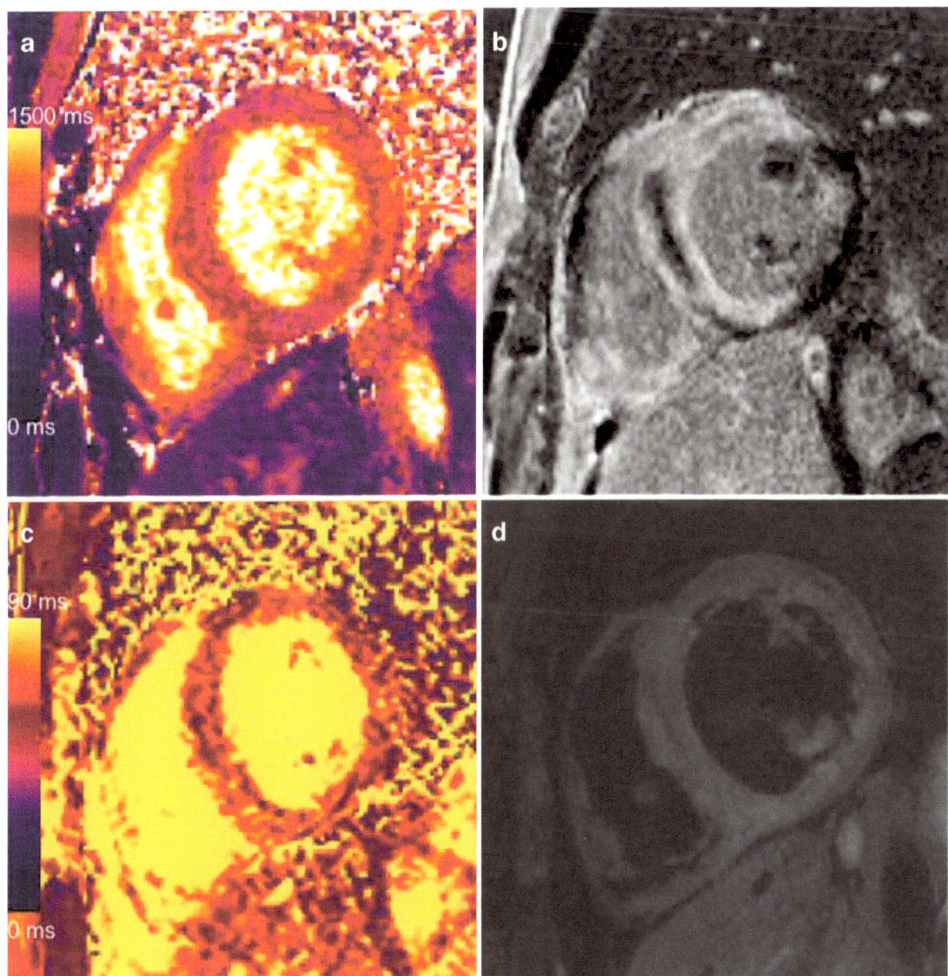

Fig. 8.6 32-year-old male with pulmonary and cardiac sarcoid who presented with malignant ventricular tachycardia. The patient subsequently had an ICD implanted. Mid-ventricular short-axis non-contrast T1 map (**a**) demonstrates a mildly elevated mean T1 value of 1050 ms (MOLLI, 1.5T). Mid short-axis LGE image (**b**) demonstrates extensive, nodular, predominantly mid-wall delayed enhancement involving both ventricles. Mid short-axis T2 map (**c**) demonstrates prolonged myocardial T2 values (55–60 ms), indicative of myocardial edema. Mid short-axis T2-weighted black blood imaged (**d**) demonstrates patchy myocardial hyperintensity in keeping with edema. 18F-FDG PET image (**e**) following adequate myocardial glucose suppression demonstrates marked abnormal myocardial uptake involving both ventricles, in keeping with inflammation. Coronal CT image confirms the presence of classic mediastinal and hilar lymphadenopathy (**f**)

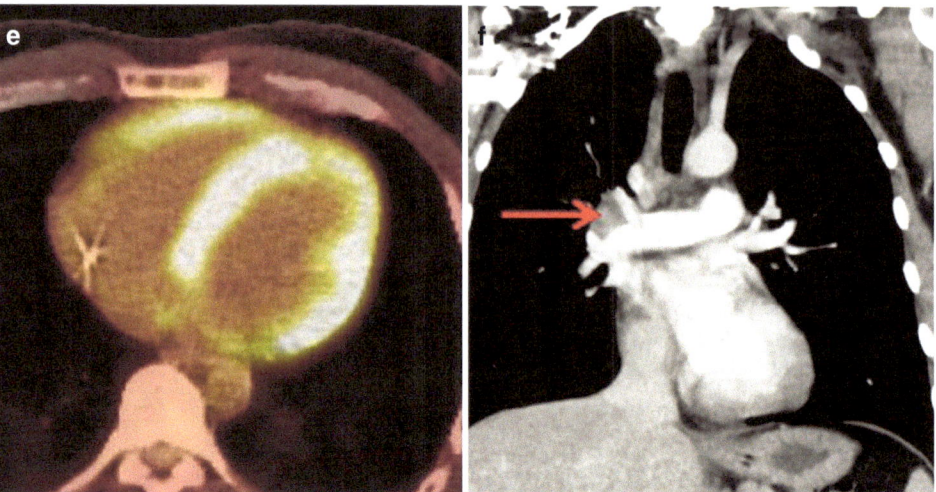

Fig. 8.6 (continued)

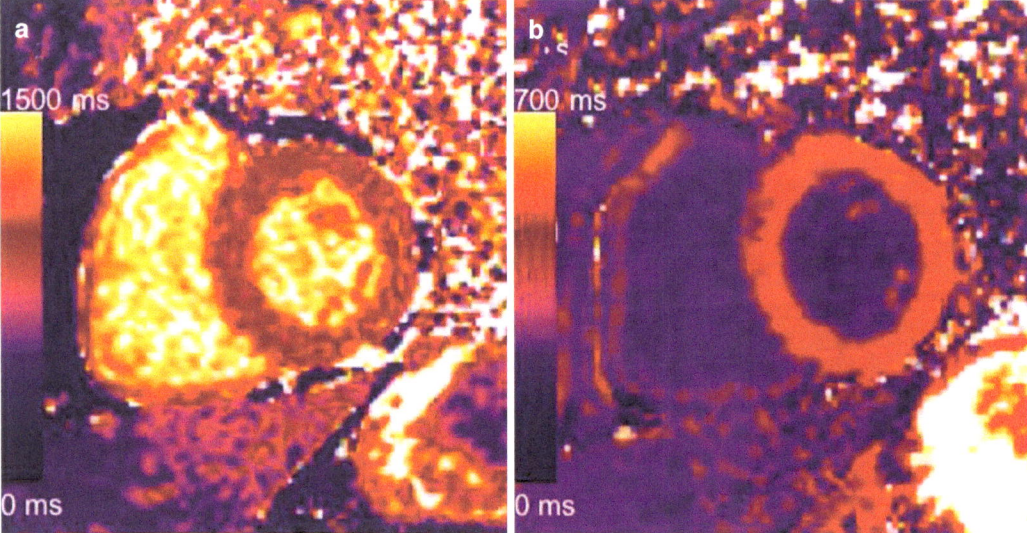

Fig. 8.7 53-year-old male with pulmonary sarcoid without cardiac involvement. Basal short-axis non-contrast T1 map (**a**) demonstrates a mean T1 value of 956 ms, within the limits of normal (MOLLI, 1.5T). Basal short-axis post-contrast T1 map (**b**) demonstrates a mean T1 value of 409 ms. Basal short-axis ECV map (**c**) demonstrates a mean global ECV value of 26%. Basal short-axis LGE image (**d**) demonstrates thin linear high-attenuation at the basal anterior septum which was favored to reflect a septal perforator

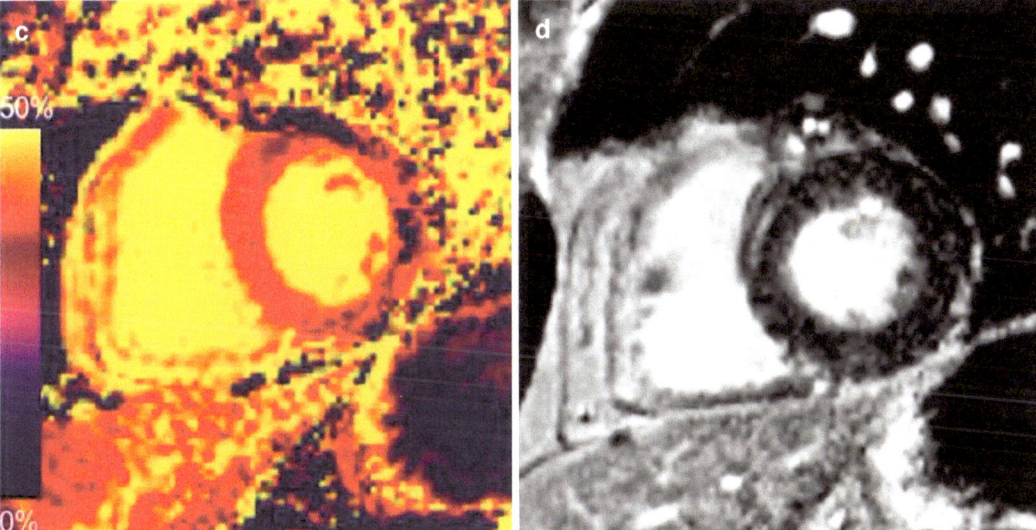

Fig. 8.7 (continued)

T1 mapping is a useful tool in the evaluation of NICM. T1 mapping findings may aid in establishing a diagnosis of NICM, monitoring response to therapy, and predicting adverse outcomes.

References

1. Maron BJ, Towbin JA, Thiene G, et al. Contemporary definitions and classification of the cardiomyopathies: an American Heart Association Scientific Statement from the Council on Clinical Cardiology, Heart Failure and Transplantation Committee; Quality of Care and Outcomes Research and Functional Genomics and Translational Biology Interdisciplinary Working Groups; and Council on Epidemiology and Prevention. Circulation. 2006;113(14):1807–16.
2. Parsai C, O'Hanlon R, Prasad SK, Mohiaddin RH. Diagnostic and prognostic value of cardiovascular magnetic resonance in non-ischaemic cardiomyopathies. J Cardiovasc Magn Reson. 2012;14:54.
3. Swift AJ, Rajaram S, Capener D, et al. LGE patterns in pulmonary hypertension do not impact overall mortality. JACC Cardiovasc Imaging. 2014;7(12):1209–17.
4. Freed BH, Gomberg-Maitland M, Chandra S, et al. Late gadolinium enhancement cardiovascular magnetic resonance predicts clinical worsening in patients with pulmonary hypertension. J Cardiovasc Magn Reson. 2012;14:11.
5. Azevedo CF, Nigri M, Higuchi ML, et al. Prognostic significance of myocardial fibrosis quantification by histopathology and magnetic resonance imaging in patients with severe aortic valve disease. J Am Coll Cardiol. 2010;56(4):278–87.
6. Baksi AJ, Pennell DJ. T1 mapping in heart failure: from technique to prognosis, toward altering outcome. Circ Cardiovasc Imaging. 2013;6(6):861–3.
7. Roujol S, Weingartner S, Foppa M, et al. Accuracy, precision, and reproducibility of four T1 mapping sequences: a head-to-head comparison of MOLLI, ShMOLLI, SASHA, and SAPPHIRE. Radiology. 2014;272(3):683–9.
8. Flett AS, Hayward MP, Ashworth MT, et al. Equilibrium contrast cardiovascular magnetic resonance for the measurement of diffuse myocardial fibrosis: preliminary validation in humans. Circulation. 2010;122(2):138–44.
9. Burt JR, Zimmerman SL, Kamel IR, Halushka M, Bluemke DA. Myocardial T1 mapping: techniques and potential applications. Radiographics. 2014;34(2):377–95.
10. Dass S, Suttie JJ, Piechnik SK, et al. Myocardial tissue characterization using magnetic resonance noncontrast t1 mapping in hypertrophic and dilated cardiomyopathy. Circ Cardiovasc Imaging. 2012;5(6):726–33.
11. Sado DM, Maestrini V, Piechnik SK, et al. Noncontrast myocardial T1 mapping using cardiovascular magnetic resonance for iron overload. J Magn Reson Imaging. 2015;41(6):1505–11.

12. Germain P, Ghannudi El S, Jeung M-Y, et al. Native T1 mapping of the heart—a pictorial review. Clin Med Insights Cardiol. 2014;8(Suppl 4):1–11.

13. Pedersen SF, Thrysøe SA, Robich MP, et al. Assessment of intramyocardial hemorrhage by T1-weighted cardiovascular magnetic resonance in reperfused acute myocardial infarction. J Cardiovasc Magn Reson. 2012;14(1):1–8.

14. Pica S, Sado DM, Maestrini V, et al. Reproducibility of native myocardial T1 mapping in the assessment of Fabry disease and its role in early detection of cardiac involvement by cardiovascular magnetic resonance. J Cardiovasc Magn Reson. 2014;16:99.

15. Germain DP. Fabry disease. Orphanet J Rare Dis. 2010;5(1):1–49.

16. Mehta A, Clarke JTR, Giugliani R, et al. Natural course of Fabry disease: changing pattern of causes of death in FOS—Fabry Outcome Survey. J Med Genet. 2009;46(8):548–52.

17. Hughes DA, Elliott PM, Shah J, et al. Effects of enzyme replacement therapy on the cardiomyopathy of Anderson-Fabry disease: a randomised, double-blind, placebo-controlled clinical trial of agalsidase alfa. Heart. 2008;94(2):153–8.

18. De Cobelli F, Esposito A, Belloni E, et al. Delayed-enhanced cardiac MRI for differentiation of Fabry's disease from symmetric hypertrophic cardiomyopathy. AJR Am J Roentgenol. 2009;192(3):W97–W102.

19. Deva DP, Hanneman K, Li Q, et al. CMR demonstration of multiple morphological phenotypes in Anderson-Fabry disease. J Cardiovasc Magn Reson. 2015;17(Suppl 1):Q68.

20. Sado DM, White SK, Piechnik SK, et al. Identification and assessment of Anderson-Fabry disease by cardiovascular magnetic resonance noncontrast myocardial T1 mapping. Circ Cardiovasc Imaging. 2013;6(3):392–8.

21. Thompson RB, Chow K, Khan A, et al. T1 mapping with cardiovascular mri is highly sensitive for Fabry disease independent of hypertrophy and sex. Circ Cardiovasc Imaging. 2013;6(5):637–45.

22. Pagano JJ, Chow K, Khan A, et al. Reduced Right ventricular native myocardial T1 in Anderson-Fabry disease: comparison to pulmonary hypertension and healthy controls. PLoS One. 2016;11(6):e0157565.

23. Sado DM, Flett AS, Banypersad SM, et al. Cardiovascular magnetic resonance measurement of myocardial extracellular volume in health and disease. Heart. 2012;98(19):1436–41.

24. Elleder M, Bradová V, Smíd F, et al. Cardiocyte storage and hypertrophy as a sole manifestation of Fabry's disease. Virchows Arch A Pathol Anat Histopathol. 1990;417(5):449–55.

25. Niemann M, Herrmann S, Hu K, et al. Differences in Fabry cardiomyopathy between female and male patients: consequences for diagnostic assessment. JACC Cardiovasc Imaging. 2011;4(6):592–601.

26. Olivieri NF, Nathan DG, MacMillan JH, et al. Survival in medically treated patients with homozygous beta-thalassemia. N Engl J Med. 1994;331(9):574–8.

27. Anderson LJ, Holden S, Davis B, et al. Cardiovascular T2-star (T2*) magnetic resonance for the early diagnosis of myocardial iron overload. Eur Heart J. 2001;22(23):2171–9.

28. Carpenter J-P, He T, Kirk P, et al. On T2* magnetic resonance and cardiac iron. Circulation. 2011;123(14):1519–28.

29. Kirk P, He T, Anderson LJ, et al. International reproducibility of single breathhold T2* MR for cardiac and liver iron assessment among five thalassemia centers. J Magn Reson Imaging. 2010;32(2):315–9.

30. Kirk P, Roughton M, Porter JB, et al. Cardiac T2* magnetic resonance for prediction of cardiac complications in thalassemia major. Circulation. 2009;120(20):1961–8.

31. Modell B, Khan M, Darlison M, Westwood MA, Ingram D, Pennell DJ. Improved survival of thalassaemia major in the UK and relation to T2* cardiovascular magnetic resonance. J Cardiovasc Magn Reson. 2008;10:42.

32. Meloni A, Positano V, Keilberg P, et al. Feasibility, reproducibility, and reliability for the T*2 iron evaluation at 3 T in comparison with 1.5 T. Magn Reson Med. 2012;68(2):543–51.

33. Wood JC. Cardiac iron determines cardiac T2*, T2, and T1 in the gerbil model of iron cardiomyopathy. Circulation. 2005;112(4):535–43.

34. Feng Y, He T, Carpenter J-P, et al. In vivo comparison of myocardial T1 with T2 and T2* in thalassaemia major. J Magn Reson Imaging. 2013;38(3):588–93.

35. Hanneman K, Nguyen ET, Thavendiranathan P, et al. Quantification of myocardial extracellular volume fraction with cardiac MR imaging in thalassemia major. Radiology. 2016;279(3):720–30.

36. Alam MH, Auger D, Smith GC, et al. T1 at 1.5T and 3T compared with conventional T2* at 1.5T for cardiac siderosis. J Cardiovasc Magn Reson. 2015;17:102.

37. Camargo GC, Rothstein T, Junqueira FP, et al. Myocardial iron quantification using modified Look-Locker inversion recovery (MOLLI) T1 mapping at 3 Tesla. J Cardiovasc Magn Reson. 2013;15(1):1–2.

38. Rapezzi C, Merlini G, Quarta CC, et al. Systemic cardiac amyloidoses: disease profiles and clinical courses of the 3 main types. Circulation. 2009;120(13):1203–12.

39. Rahman JE, Helou EF, Gelzer-Bell R, et al. Noninvasive diagnosis of biopsy-proven cardiac amyloidosis. J Am Coll Cardiol. 2004;43(3):410–5.

40. Syed IS, Glockner JF, Feng D, et al. Role of cardiac magnetic resonance imaging in the detection of cardiac amyloidosis. JACC Cardiovasc Imaging. 2010;3(2):155–64.

41. Vogelsberg H, Mahrholdt H, Deluigi CC, et al. Cardiovascular magnetic resonance in clinically suspected cardiac amyloidosis: noninvasive imaging compared to endomyocardial biopsy. J Am Coll Cardiol. 2008;51(10):1022–30.

42. Karamitsos TD, Piechnik SK, Banypersad SM, et al. Noncontrast T1 mapping for the diagnosis of

cardiac amyloidosis. JACC Cardiovasc Imaging. 2013;6(4):488–97.

43. Hosch W, Bock M, Libicher M, et al. MR-relaxometry of myocardial tissue: significant elevation of T1 and T2 relaxation times in cardiac amyloidosis. Investig Radiol. 2007;42(9):636–42.

44. Fontana M, Banypersad SM, Treibel TA, et al. Native T1 mapping in transthyretin amyloidosis. JACC Cardiovasc Imaging. 2014;7(2):157–65.

45. Banypersad SM, Sado DM, Flett AS, et al. Quantification of myocardial extracellular volume fraction in systemic AL amyloidosis: an equilibrium contrast cardiovascular magnetic resonance study. Circ Cardiovasc Imaging. 2013;6(1):34–9.

46. Banypersad SM, Fontana M, Maestrini V, et al. T1 mapping and survival in systemic light-chain amyloidosis. Eur Heart J. 2015;36(4):244–51.

47. Rybicki BA, Major M, Popovich JJ, Maliarik MJ, Iannuzzi MC. Racial differences in sarcoidosis incidence: a 5-year study in a health maintenance organization. Am J Epidemiol. 1997;145(3):234–41.

48. Iannuzzi MC, Rybicki BA, Teirstein AS. Sarcoidosis. N Engl J Med. 2007;357(21):2153–65.

49. Newman LS, Rose CS, Maier LA. Sarcoidosis. N Engl J Med. 1997;336(17):1224–34.

50. Silverman KJ, Hutchins GM, Bulkley BH. Cardiac sarcoid: a clinicopathologic study of 84 unselected patients with systemic sarcoidosis. Circulation. 1978;58(6):1204–11.

51. Perry A, Vuitch F. Causes of death in patients with sarcoidosis. A morphologic study of 38 autopsies with clinicopathologic correlations. Arch Pathol Lab Med. 1995;119(2):167–72.

52. Vignaux O. Cardiac sarcoidosis: spectrum of MRI features. Am J Roentgenol. 2005;184(1):249–54.

53. Uemura A, Morimoto S, Hiramitsu S, Kato Y, Ito T, Hishida H. Histologic diagnostic rate of cardiac sarcoidosis: evaluation of endomyocardial biopsies. Am Heart J. 1999;138(2 Pt 1):299–302.

54. Patel MR, Cawley PJ, Heitner JF, et al. Detection of myocardial damage in patients with sarcoidosis. Circulation. 2009;120(20):1969–77.

55. Vignaux O, Dhote R, Duboc D, et al. Detection of myocardial involvement in patients with sarcoidosis applying T2-weighted, contrast-enhanced, and cine magnetic resonance imaging: initial results of a prospective study. J Comput Assist Tomogr. 2002;26(5):762–7.

56. Smedema J-P, Snoep G, van Kroonenburgh MPG, et al. Evaluation of the accuracy of gadolinium-enhanced cardiovascular magnetic resonance in the diagnosis of cardiac sarcoidosis. J Am Coll Cardiol. 2005;45(10):1683–90.

57. Youssef G, Leung E, Mylonas I, et al. The use of 18F-FDG PET in the diagnosis of cardiac sarcoidosis: a systematic review and metaanalysis including the Ontario experience. J Nucl Med. 2012;53(2):241–8.

58. Okumura W, Iwasaki T, Toyama T, et al. Usefulness of fasting 18F-FDG PET in identification of cardiac sarcoidosis. J Nucl Med. 2004;45(12):1989–98.

59. Maron MS. Contrast-enhanced CMR in HCM: what lies behind the bright light of LGE and why it now matters. JACC Cardiovasc Imaging. 2013;6(5):597–9.

60. Moravsky G, Ofek E, Rakowski H, et al. Myocardial fibrosis in hypertrophic cardiomyopathy: accurate reflection of histopathological findings by CMR. JACC Cardiovasc Imaging. 2013;6(5):587–96.

61. Moon JCC, Reed E, Sheppard MN, et al. The histologic basis of late gadolinium enhancement cardiovascular magnetic resonance in hypertrophic cardiomyopathy. J Am Coll Cardiol. 2004;43(12):2260–4.

62. Serra JJ, Monte GU, Mello ES, et al. Images in cardiovascular medicine. Cardiac sarcoidosis evaluated by delayed-enhanced magnetic resonance imaging. Circulation. 2003;107(20):e188–9.

63. Wu TJ, Ong JJ, Hwang C, et al. Characteristics of wave fronts during ventricular fibrillation in human hearts with dilated cardiomyopathy: role of increased fibrosis in the generation of reentry. J Am Coll Cardiol. 1998;32(1):187–96.

64. Yamagishi H, Shirai N, Takagi M, et al. Identification of cardiac sarcoidosis with (13)N-NH(3)/(18)F-FDG PET. J Nucl Med. 2003;44(7):1030–6.

65. Hoey ETD, Gulati GS, Ganeshan A, Watkin RW, Simpson H, Sharma S. Cardiovascular MRI for assessment of infectious and inflammatory conditions of the heart. Am J Roentgenol. 2011;197(1):103–12.

66. Friedrich MG, Sechtem U, Schulz-Menger J, et al. Cardiovascular magnetic resonance in myocarditis: a JACC white paper. J Am Coll Cardiol. 2009;53(17):1475–87.

67. Thavendiranathan P, Walls M, Giri S, et al. Improved detection of myocardial involvement in acute inflammatory cardiomyopathies using T2 mapping. Circ Cardiovasc Imaging. 2012;5(1):102–10.

68. Crouser ED, Ono C, Tran T, He X, Raman SV. Improved detection of cardiac sarcoidosis using magnetic resonance with myocardial T2 mapping. Am J Respir Crit Care Med. 2014;189(1):109–12.

69. Ferreira VM, Piechnik SK, Dall'Armellina E, et al. T(1) mapping for the diagnosis of acute myocarditis using CMR: comparison to T2-weighted and late gadolinium enhanced imaging. JACC Cardiovasc Imaging. 2013;6(10):1048–58.

70. Ferreira VM, Piechnik SK, Dall'Armellina E, et al. Native T1-mapping detects the location, extent and patterns of acute myocarditis without the need for gadolinium contrast agents. J Cardiovasc Magn Reson. 2014;16(1):1–11.

71. Puntmann VO, D'Cruz D, Smith Z, et al. Native myocardial T1 mapping by cardiovascular magnetic resonance imaging in subclinical cardiomyopathy in patients with systemic lupus erythematosus. Circ Cardiovasc Imaging. 2013;6(2):295–301.